Impossible... Or So They Said

A Stem Cell Experience Lived
And Written By

Shawn C. Wickard

COPYRIGHT

ISBN-13: 978-1518884641

ISBN-10: 1518884644

I would like to dedicate this book and thank the many Doctors, Researchers, Nurses, and other staff that made my experience at the National Institutes of Health so memorable.

There are many others to thank for their help in editing, polishing and otherwise shaping the contents of this book such as Todd Wickard, Melissa Western, Stephanie Cannon and many others.

I also need to thank my original physical therapists Jason Terry and Stephanie Obradovich for teaching me to walk the final time.

My Personal Trainer Surba Tucker for seeing what is possible even before I caught the vision.

Contents

Taking The Bull By The Horns, Or In This Case A Ram

When I was 18, I had the opportunity with several friends to help a neighbor out by taking down some fencing. This wasn't ordinary fencing. It enclosed a piece of land where he kept several exotic animals. Among them were an aoudad ram (Barbary ram) and a black buck antelope. This ram had trophy sized horns similar to the logo used for Dodge trucks, the horns of the antelope were long straight spirals and about two feet long.

When we arrived we were met by Skip Clemens, a true Grizzly Adams in appearance and lifestyle. He was my neighbor and friend. In addition to Skip a couple of Seattle's Woodland Park Zoo officials were also in the pen. We were told, though, the ram had been darted several times with tranquilizers so that he could be moved to a new property on the other side of town, yet none of the tranquilizers had subdued the animal.

They needed a volunteer.

Have you ever watch movies where there is a lineup of volunteers and one is asked to step forward and the rest of the line simultaneously steps backwards? Yea, I was the one left out in front.

I entered the pen and closed the gate. I was instructed by one of the officials that they were going to guide the ram through parallel lines of brush so that this animal would be somewhat guided as he ran towards me. I nervously chuckled, yea right. He then told me to grab him by the horns and wrestle him down to the ground, kind of like what you see at a rodeo when the cowboy brings down the calf to rope his hooves. As we were walking towards our designated positions he then instructed me to NOT release my grip on the ram once I had him. I naively asked why not, "Because he will kill you", he answered.

If I wasn't a little nervous up till this time I was now full blown wishing I was somewhere else! Who in their right mind would want to be in the same pen as a mountain ram that stood just a little shorter than my 5 foot 10!!

As the animal began rushing toward me down this little natural chute I nervously shifted weight from side to side with my arms slightly bent in anticipation of grabbing him.

When he was about to reach me I grabbed those horns of his, one in each hand and thrust his head to my left and down, using his momentum to bring him to the ground. With a grunt and an exclamation of excitement and nervousness I began to be proud of myself for wrestling this huge wild animal to the ground.

I had captured a ram by myself with my own bare hands I thought!!

As I looked up I found the other zoo officials draped all over this animal subduing him and tying up his hoofs like a cowboy does to a calf. I was slightly disappointed that I didn't really capture him single handed but I certainly was the key to capturing him.

Life comes at you fast. What I learned that day was to be prepared for life to change in an instant. When I was first struck with numbness and eventually paralysis, I felt a lot like I did the day this ram was steered towards me. I had to grab hold and ride it out to the end. Life comes at you fast and you do not always have time to prepare a reaction. You go with your gut instinct and hope for the best. It was all I could do. The doctors didn't know what was going on and when they finally did they didn't have any answers as to why and what to expect. I was literally on my own.

Character cannot be developed in ease and quiet. Only through experience of trial and suffering can the soul be strengthened, ambition inspired, and success achieved.

Helen Keller

Waking Up Is A Gamble

I awoke on an overcast gray Sunday morning on the 22nd of February 1998 to an icy type burning feeling in my legs from the shins down. I was 27 years old. I thought perhaps I had slept wrong and maybe kinked my back or neck in some weird way. I went to church and kept wondering why I was feeling this odd sensation. Regardless of what I did, the burning feeling persisted. Nothing seemed to change throughout the day although it was only a low level burning sensation.

Later that afternoon a new feeling started in the middle of my back. In between my shoulder blades was a gradual swelling feeling that became extremely uncomfortable. Later that night this area emanated quite a bit of pain, no matter what position I slept in, the swelling pressure spread from my shoulder blades to my spine and I could not do anything to stop the pain. I did not sleep a wink that night, while tossing and turning the whole night.

After work the next day, I went to the chiropractor thinking I had tweaked my back, or neck. The chiropractor worked on my back and

I went home. I didn't feel any better that night or the next day. By Wednesday, I was fully numb from the chest down and about 50% weaker.

That Wednesday afternoon I made an interesting discovery about numbness as I approached the back of my Jeep Wrangler I heard a loud thud and felt something solid against the front of my leg. I had struck the trailer hitch with my shin in full stride! I looked down, pulled up my pant leg, and immediately saw a quarter inch deep dent in the middle of my shin! I let out a huge sigh as I realized I did not feel a thing. What would have normally brought me to tears had hardly fazed me. That was my first experience learning the up side to not feeling anything in my legs.

Despite how cool it was to do so much damage to a shin and not feeling any pain, I was worried about what was happening. Yet, I shrugged it off as no big deal and thought that it would soon go away. I never considered the possibility that the pain and numbness could lead to something worse.

At this point I was very concerned about what was happening. I had made an appointment with a neurologist for the afternoon of the 25th. After the exam, which was pretty basic, she made an appointment at the hospital for an MRI for Friday afternoon. I arrived at 3 p.m. for the 3:30 p.m. MRI. I undressed and slipped into the hospital pants and shirt that are required. After the MRI, as I was getting dressed the radiologist came in to talk to me.

I have to say I was quite amused at his face as he came in. You know in the movies or television shows when the scene has a doctor about to give some really sad depressing news to the patient and their family? He had that face and demeanor as he said that he normally doesn't talk to the patients first without the doctor but since none were around he came in to tell me that there were some inconsistencies in my MRI of the spine and that he wanted me to get a brain scan also. I asked if I should schedule the appointment for some time soon and he replied that I was going back in right then. I was thinking, "This must be serious, huh!"

After the brain MRI he told me to check in with the emergency room and to get some further testing done. I checked in and found a seat while I called a friend; we had planned to have dinner that evening. I told her things needed to change and that I was in the emergency room, waiting to see a doctor. She went to the restaurant we had planned to eat at, (one of my favorite Mexican restaurants) and brought me some dinner.

Once I was called back, to the treatment area of the emergency room it is all a blur. I ended up getting a spinal tap which is a test where a needle is inserted in between your lower vertebrae into the spinal sack/canal and spinal fluid is drawn out with a syringe. They had drugged me with something that really made me feel great, and no pain. I was extremely groggy upon waking after the procedure. My friend had to drive me home since they wouldn't let me drive home alone. By that time it was 1:30 in the morning. My 90 minute appointment had lasted for almost 11 hours.

The next day, Saturday the 28th, I drove to Park City, Utah with some friends to meet for lunch. I could barely shuffle my feet and was really having a difficult lifting my feet off the ground. I learned how much this hurt when I had to walk down a steep flight of steps to the bathroom. I barely made it down, but going back up was a different story entirely. I could barely make my leg raise my foot much higher than the step I was trying to clear. In that moment the number of steps seemed daunting and I would not get back up the staircase.

That evening I went to meet with a couple of friends for dinner. While I was waiting for them to show up I saw a couple of other friends out in the parking lot and we started chatting. As we did I began to have trouble getting air into my lungs. Just about that time my friends showed up and it was quickly decided that they were going to take me to the hospital again. I couldn't breathe and I began to hyperventilate. I'm sure my fear wasn't helping me much. I was truly scared; this lack of control frightened me.

I ended up being admitted to the hospital for what ended up being an 8 day stay. This was also my first stay in a hospital. I remember calling my father and telling him what was going on, I knew he'd understand as he was living on a kidney dialysis machine due to kidney failure years earlier. The next week was a bit of a blur and I only remember a few things. I was having pain in my abdomen and had a standing order for Demerol to alleviate that pain. A couple of gals were visiting and I shifted my position in the bed and all of a sudden that pain became unbearable. I sat on the edge of the bed while I rubbed my bare foot on the carpeted floor to draw the pain away in a vain attempt to lessen it.

Also, because the pain grew so rapidly in its intensity, I began to swear in my favorite choice words. It was sometimes in a soft whisper but when the pain crescendoed so would the words and how loud they were. The nurse finally gave me the Demerol and the pain began to alleviate. As that was happening I discovered that a girl who I was friends with but also was quite taken by came in. She had been standing outside the door as the swearing had taken place. I was embarrassed and apologized completely for that display but she luckily was okay with it and understood because she could hear how much pain I was in.

She sat and talked with me as I fell in and out of consciousness for several hours. I have always appreciated that kind act. It really made a difference to me there was someone present while I was feeling significant pain and acted like a true friend to me that night.

I had a doctor come up the next day after a test and began by saying he can see why I was in so much pain. I had two duodenal ulcers, which is in the tube leading from the stomach to the intestines, and they were huge. I got set up on meds and I began to feel much better.

I was released on the following Saturday. A friend had me over from the hospital so I didn't have to go home right away and while I was extremely weak it was a fun afternoon and evening. A mutual friend of ours drove me home since one, I couldn't drive, and two, there was no family available since my grandma, who I lived with, was in St. George all week. I lived in the basement and that was a big decision maker. How do I make sure when I get down there I don't have to come back up for anything. I was able to make it down and sleep in my own bed that night. It felt so good to do that. The best healing comes when you're rested in your own bed!

That afternoon grandma came home with my aunt, her husband, and her two kids. Not a single one of them understood or tried to understand that it wasn't my muscles but my nerves that were the problem. The nerves were the reason why I went numb and weak. It wasn't going to be a 'just go to the gym' and work the muscles out kind of recovery. It was extremely frustrating to have to even try and convince them that this was beyond my control and that recovery might be my choice but there was no choice how quickly I got there.

This not only annoyed me, it hurt me. It hurt my feelings that no one was trying to at least understand that there was something terribly wrong and I needed a little support. I believed "family" would at least try to be empathetic to what I and the doctors couldn't understand nor explain as a show of support. Why do I need to even convince "family" that I am simply sick and need more than a little help? I would learn that they simply did not have a mindset that could grasp what I was going through. They couldn't even come up with the questions to ask in order to understand. Even if they stumbled or at least tried I could have understood the difficulty in understanding something so medically odd. But, at least give a damn. This frustrated me more than anything. I felt on the defensive when explaining what was happening.

People are always blaming their circumstances for what they are. I don't believe in circumstances. The people who get on in this world are the people who get up and look for the circumstances they want, and if they can't find them, make them

George Bernard Shaw

Visualize The End Results – (Im)Possible Principle

I used to drive the course of a race to determine my strategy. I would drive the entire course so I had no question of its path. I would go to bed and lie there picturing every move I planned on making the next morning. When I awoke I didn't think anymore, I acted. It was ingrained in my very soul.

Living our lives deliberately and purposefully allows us to work towards the end results. When we do this all of our actions will lead to the end goal just like driving the race course the night before. By having a clear vision of what we are working towards each of our steps become a part of the process.

So must we make our efforts deliberate and planned while leaving plenty of room for the unanticipated to occur. With the picture painted of our path we can make adjustments as needed without taking ourselves off the intended path.

I first learned this technique in high school. I ran track and cross country and we were taught how to lie down and picture the race we planned on executing. It wasn't very clear at first. In fact it was more of a short nap than anything productive. As I practiced visualization, the clearer I was able to picture the type of race I wished to run. The more I did this, the more I could actually run the race I had begun to visualize. The technique teaches us the power of suggestion. We each have the ability to live our desired lives by learning to picture the outcome first and then learning to execute it.

This is how I believe I learned to picture myself healing. I visualized stronger legs. I pictured the activities I wished to continue to enjoy and I set out to make it happen as I had visualized it.

So, I'll Be Fine, Yea?

I began my recovery by going to see a chiropractor first. He happened to have a multidisciplinary office and a physical therapist was in the back office. We had to speak and come up with a plan of action as my spine couldn't be manipulated since my spinal cord was actually swollen. That is what the MRI showed. I didn't know the spinal cord could swell. Therefore, any rotating of my spine could permanently damage it and I could be left with permanent disabilities. Once we came up with a plan we got to work. That 8 days in the hospital had rendered my muscles so atrophied that my back was thrown out of alignment by just leaning over the counter brushing my teeth and caused me a great deal of discomfort. Not only were the muscles in my back atrophied but my legs were still extraordinarily weak.

Once I began physical therapy my stated goal was to hike Fiery Furnace in Arches National Park outside Moab, Utah. I was heading there in 2 months with a group and that was my favorite hike. In fact, it was the only hike I was ever interested in down there. It is a series of slot canyons almost stacked upon one another rising probably 100

15

feet in height or more. They are somewhat interconnected but not in a clearly defined path.

The beginning of the hike is a path that leads in but soon it gives way to a muddied area of rock and cryptobiotic soil. This is soil that is alive. It has a crusty surface and if you leave a footprint in it will stay that way for hundreds of years. It is something that you're advised to not step in at all when watching the video during the permitting process. The pathway is strewn with boulders of varying sizes in piles along the way as well as solid rock. The goal is to choose a pathway based upon your assessment of the loose rocks, solid rock and to use these as your footing. I love the meandering pathways of these slot canyons and the myriad ways one can maneuver through them piecing together a hike of majestic quality.

This is an awesome hike and I made the goal to get my legs built up in strength for this hike. I worked out twice a week during these two months with two therapists in building my strength with exercises and weight training and walking on a treadmill. All of this training combined, slowly built my strength up to probably 80-85% of what it was before the numbness and weakness set in. As I hiked, I thoroughly enjoyed myself and even though it was a much tougher hike than normal. It tested my endurance, but I accomplished my goal. I felt a sense of completion afterward.

The rest of the summer and fall went by without too much excitement and I mentally felt the whole thing was a glitch and I was only looking at the future. I moved out of grandma's that August; it was a good deal to live rent free; but she asked me to move, or rather she suggested that it wasn't working out having me live there she felt it was perhaps, time for me to find a new place to live. I moved in with a friend that summer and things were going great in an awesome bachelor's pad. We had a creek in the back yard with an old pond that even had a waterfall in it, and a large yard. It was the best place I've ever lived for the mere ability to relax and enjoy life a little. We had some awesome BBQ's that summer and things seemed to be looking up.

One who gains strength by overcoming obstacles possesses the only strength which can overcome adversity.

Albert Sweitzer

FUBAR

When I was 12 my siblings and I spent the Memorial weekend at my aunt and uncle's. They lived about 30-40 minutes from us at the time and it seemed like a world away for me. We did what cousins would do, we played, we goofed off and we stayed up way late watching shows we weren't supposed to on cable television. It was a fun weekend. We got home on Monday only to be herded into the family room to be told by our mother that our father was in the hospital and that he was very ill. We were told that we would be going to the hospital to visit him. A lot of thoughts began speeding through my mind. What exactly was wrong, what does this mean, do we get our father back?

When we reached his room I purposefully stayed in the doorway. Somehow actually going in meant some sort of commitment I wasn't ready for. I observed silently and saw that he had several tubes sticking out of him and yet he seemed to be in a decent enough mood. What we were then told was his kidneys were operating at 15%. He needed a transplant or else he would be on a dialysis machine the rest of his life.

He eventually decided to go the dialysis machine route. This meant he was hooked up to a machine that would extract his blood which was run through a series of filters in order to clean it of the impurities that our kidneys usually perform before bringing the cleaned blood back to his body. This took anywhere from 3-4 hours a session and he had to do this 3-4 days a week for the rest of his life. Each of us were given a chance to go in to the clinic with him and experience a dialysis treatment. I hated it. I cannot put into words how much this negatively impacted me. I couldn't stand seeing him hooked up to this machine, I couldn't stand the two tubes sticking out of both his arms. One for the blood to flow to the machine and one that took it back to his body. I vowed that day to never step into a hospital again.

Too bad I couldn't keep that vow.

From that moment on I felt like I was the man of the house therefore I personally shouldered that level of responsibility. Whether this was implied implicitly or it was explicit I do not remember but I did feel like I needed to step up. I of course didn't know what this meant at the time and to be honest I still don't. It was rough on us as a family and I now truly feel this was the beginning of the end for us as a cohesive unit. Nothing was the same after this. I stopped having a father figure that was involved and there for me to share with me how to function in the world as an adult. I lost a father who could go camping with me and instruct me in those lessons I would utilize as an adult. I felt I lost something irreplaceable and things were never the same. I felt alone on my journey from then on.

Life seemed to coast in a haze from there. No direction. No guidance as to the changing of life for me as I entered my formative teenage years. Listless doesn't quite cover it but close. Happiness wasn't found at home for me. It was very rough. The slow falling apart began almost immediately. The parents were so worried about my father's health that all the children took a back seat in priority. Granted we all wanted him to be in full and complete health if you asked us back then but we each had our own needs that needed to be paid attention to. I feel looking back that because of this gap in attention we each began to realize that we needed to fill that void ourselves in our own manner. I spent more and more time outside with my next door neighbor Dave Scott playing in the woods behind our house. In the summer time I could be gone from sunup to sundown without any questions from my parents. I thought of myself as an adult when it came to how I governed myself.

I knew I was making right choices because I wasn't purposefully trying to get in trouble of any kind. The tranquility of my existence when I was forming my own world outside of my house was shattered every night when I had to return to it. The energy between the two was drastic and polarizing. One was expansive and full of growth developing my imagination and the other seemed to cap it and even squash it.

I read a lot during this time. I once read over 250 books in my 8th grade year. We had just moved to a new area of town and I didn't know anybody in the new neighborhood so I would sometimes read a book a day. I spent a lot of time in my head when it came to reading and visiting other worlds of my own making. It allowed me to find further ways to escape my reality and I cherished reading for that very reason. School was easy for me. It didn't even challenge me so I was bored by it. It didn't capture my attention and imagination quite like reading books did.

It was during this time that the arguments between my parents would start at the dinner table and last until bedtime. They were explosive and conducted as if we weren't there. It seemed we were dragged as a family unit into the problems when we children should have been kept away from it and allowed to be kids. In Psychology this is referred to as role reversal or parentification. It's described as when the child is relied upon as the adult more that the adults are acting. This describes perfectly the dynamic I grew up in.

The family unit wasn't just fracturing because the adults couldn't handle their stress, there were abuses. Their lack of self-control as parents and adults handling my father's health spilled over to how they treated us as children and me as the oldest. I feel now that the lack of control that my mother may have felt lead her to an abusive path setting her as the controlling interest and that what she wanted won out over everybody else's interest. Her problems were worse than our problems. I didn't seem to exist as Shawn, the oldest son, in her eyes I existed as an entity that she could abuse because of her perception that my father was failing as a husband.

I did the best I could to survive. I coped well most days and there were a couple of instances where I broke down, not understanding why I felt so lost, neglected, and ignored. I felt unloved and unappreciated. I was an emotional mess but no one would know that about me except a few people. Even then they would not know how badly off I was because, I never opened up and I never asked for help. All the children were left to their own devices to raise themselves. I've been raising myself since I was 12 years old.

My mother, who we ended up titling el Madre, became distant and full of anger and spite. She lashed out at the closest person she could since my father was at dialysis. This left him depleted of energy and the time to be the father of the house. I was the target of this abuse. My personality was almost exactly like my father's. He didn't take crap from anybody. He and I shared that trait and I almost lost that during this time. I took a lot of abuse from her and only in the last little while have been able to acknowledge it. She used me as a proxy for her anger for him getting sick, for him not getting better, and for ruining her future. This anger was directed at me. I could do no right even though I was to act like the man of the house. There were expectations that no one could live up to yet I would be in trouble if I didn't live up to them. I was kicked out of the house once, with a long stick as she closed the garage door, hitting, poking and swiping at me until the door closed. Yelling at me to not return. She would always claim we had no money and that we were poor yet she could spend over $5,000 renovating a bathroom barely 4 feet by 10 feet in size.

For example there would be a fridge full of food yet if I ate any of it I would be beat. Just about the only food that became a mainstay for all of us was popcorn. It became my one afterschool snack that wouldn't get the smack down from her. It took the place of meals sometimes. My mother got into health food and it seemed like she was forcing us to take all these supplements in her quest to find a way to reverse my father's illness. Food became a manipulation tool for her from then on. In high school it only got worse.

As much as she touted health food and eating right she had huge stashes of candy, junk food, and other comfort foods that I would find and, of course, eat. I wasn't just starving for food, I was emotionally starving for attention. Maybe this lead to finding all the hiding places for her comfort foods and eating it to gain a little attention. Even her being angry at me is attention. I wasn't all that picky by this time. I needed what most receive from a parent but I wasn't receiving this.

The truth is I have suffered all forms of abuse at her hands such as physical, mental, emotional, verbal and sexual abuses. Some occurred when I was too young to possibly remember while most occurred every day. In the end evil will find a way to show itself. I have unknowingly been battling the side effects of these abuses my whole life. Any type of abuse is insidious and evil no matter who perpetuates them. I never sought to be a statistic or to bare my soul by writing about these things but it's best for my healing. If sharing this helps someone else learn that they too can heal from even the worst offenses brought by a parent, sibling or family friend and even a stranger then I will feel better about sharing such personal things. Only a very small handful of friends even know about this part of my past. I have barely acknowledged it to myself till recently.

I get together with one friend quite often for breakfast and she recently told of an event that I still have no memory of. Heidi, whom I've known since at least my 9th grade year was asked to come over to talk to me by a mutual friend, Rich. I apparently was in a bad way so she came over. She remembers my mom's fake smile welcoming her into our house and allowing her to go to my room where I was.

As she states it, she was uncomfortable with this since she was raised to not go into boys' rooms alone. As she walked through the kitchen which had an opening to our television room she saw my sisters looking at her with a, who are you, look. She saw my father sitting at the kitchen table in his own world sitting alone. My room was just past him.

When she entered my room I was listening to music. I pointed to the tape that was playing saying that once I was finished listening to that I intended to listen to the stack of tapes next to it and afterward I declared that I was going to kill myself. She told me there were two other times she had to talk me down from harming myself. I was lost during my junior high and high school years. I didn't realize that I was willing to take things to that extreme to escape that existence. I saw no way out and thought by leaving this earth I would be in a better place.

Existing just to exist is a living hell that far too many people live every single day. They are most likely people we know, friends we see, and family members we live with. Yet, we can be oblivious to the pain that these individuals in our lives are feeling and perhaps are seeking a permanent escape from. We need to be more like my friend Heidi in being willing to ask the hard questions, show up unexpectedly and exhibit caring for whatever that person is going through. You don't need to solve their problems. They aren't looking for that. They, I, was looking for someone to show they cared and that made all the difference for me.

As you can probably tell I don't have many memories of most if not all of my childhood. The ones I do have are not ones I wish to keep remembering. My brother whom I converse with quite often has brought things up here and there to see if I remember and I do not. From his perspective there were so many things wrong with how things were back then; I need to share them as further example of the terrible pressure that our mom placed on me and us during this time.

She had a horrible way to manipulate my father in order to beat me when he got home from dialysis, usually because I didn't succumb to her abuses. She did this technique to get the other kids beat depending on the week. She used guilt, shame, fear and obligation to get her way. She would prevent the same uncle who we were spending the weekend with when my father got sick from coming over saying it was a bad time. Thus preventing our cousins' from coming over and us have good times and cutting off the one family relation that we had outside contact with.

She would use her affection for us to make us compete for her attention, like an emperor in Rome watching the gladiator's battle for his amusement. This is ultimately what split the siblings and me from ever really having any solid relationship of any kind. We were pitted against each other without knowing it so we never have had solid sibling bonds that most other families have with each other. We were fated from the beginning it seemed from ever having any kind of loving example of what makes up a family and other wonderful attributes we needed to pass on to a new generation. Everything I was taught or shown has me never wanting my own children. If I can't heal from the illusion of lies that make up my perception of family I do not want to bring in another generation of children to experience what I did.

The examples of fighting at the dinner table throughout my junior and high school years became an example of what I never wanted to have in my future family. I am not entirely sure of the impact upon my other siblings. I am the oldest of 7, my brother then 5 sisters. I speak to my brother despite our childhood of trying to kill each other. He has a story where he had a knife to my throat wanting to use it on me, which I do not remember at all. I have a faint memory of walking to my room to end a bitter fight we were having when my hand reached out and grabbed a knife without me consciously choosing to. Prior to grabbing the knife, my brother and I were putting each other's head under our arms in a head lock to then ram it into the door frame in the kitchen. That was our last fight.

Over the last 7 years we've talked quite often with one another. As I have healed physically we have begun to address the emotional healing. We have learned from and discussed with each other the hell of our childhood and have come to terms that it wasn't us. We were the product of this but it doesn't necessarily have to define us. The rest of the sisters and I do not have much of a relationship to speak of.

When I moved out I left everyone and everything behind without looking back. I ended up moving to Idaho for college with my truck packed with all the things I wanted to take with me. I knew I wasn't coming back. I left all my siblings behind as the relationships there were too combative and too fractured to mend in those circumstances. I knew I needed to leave in order to get in a better place for me. After the last semester of college I moved on to Salt Lake City where I still reside to this day.

I spent my high school years spending as much time as I could with a trio of friends with whom I am still friends; I did everything with them. We hung out and watched movies, we went on trips to Oregon, we spent a lot of time together and in those times I felt normal and accepted as a person. Any time I spent outside of my house were great days. These times showed me that what I was living in was wrong.

I couldn't have, at the time, told you what was exactly wrong but I knew it wasn't what everyone else experienced. I could tell by the relationships of my 3 friends with their parents that they were friends with them like I was to my friends. From that example I was shown a better way to be. I became an additional son to these parents as well. We are all friends. I learned to escape my wrong parental examples and always look for the examples my friends parents gave me.

Without realizing it at the time they were giving me the correct example of how to treat family as well as friends. We treat people with love no matter who they are because we are all the same in the end. We are all trying to get through our stuff and if we can do it together than we can do it completely. It will take a lot for my siblings to get over their perceptions of what we all grew up in and to make amends to deal with it as they need to but perhaps one day there will be a semblance of a family unit again in this life.

The abuse I endured left no visible scars but the impact of it is felt every day as I face it and separate myself from it. Since then I have researched and now understand the connection of negative emotions and disease. It seems obvious now but I could not have seen the connection then. Stress in whatever form is debilitating to our bodies. Science in recent months and years have begun to recognize that around 80% of our diseases have a stress component to them. Naturally we think of work stress, traffic stress, or money stress as the things we face daily. But abuse is also stress. It may be traumatic but it is still stress. It needs to be directed somewhere. It may take years to manifest itself but it is still stress and it will have horrible effects upon our health.

I have read books by authors who research this connection and who in their own way make the connections of negative emotion to our physical health very apparent and real. This has allowed me to further explore healing, past the physical one that I would experience later on and delve into healing myself from within. It has been a powerful journey that has allowed me to find comfort in my own skin and to learn to appreciate what it is I have been through and to learn to be happy from within despite that past.

Years later when I myself became ill and became a frequent visitor of the hospitals I would reflect upon the one life lesson my father unintentionally taught me. When you go through hard times you put your head down and you keep moving forward. It is important to do that no matter what. You put up with the lack of comfort. You put up with the pain. You keep trudging forward.

Because there is no backwards.

It's weird that this is the one life lesson I couldn't have known I needed and it has become my bedrock. I am full of gratitude now as I look back in time and see his example to me on how to not settle for the answers of today but to seek resolution for tomorrow. This is what fuels my drive to heal from this abusive past. It made me who I am today and it gave me the foundation to be able to handle and survive the medical problems I ended up having. While I wish I could have had a different childhood and experience, I simply have to look forward to the day I can start my own family, this time armed with a healed heart for the family I will have in the future.

The only thing worse than being blind is having no sight and no vision.

Do You Believe In Déjà Vu?

October 9, 1998 I awoke and the numbness and weakness both came back. It hit hard and fast this time. I was devastated. I felt lost. Only this time I felt there was nowhere to turn. I was on my own. And it felt in more ways than one this time. It felt complete. I don't know how to explain that feeling but I knew it was going to get worse.

Instead of spending time in the hospital my doctor set me up with home health care and once the nurse comes in and gets an I.V. started I was on my own in giving myself the SoluMedrol, or liquid prednisone steroids. I had my own portable I.V. pole and everything. This drug was an anti-inflammatory that would reduce the swelling of my spinal cord. It is a great drug for that but it is a nasty drug in 99 other ways. I hated to be on this drug. It caused you to feel odd and it made you feel swollen or bloated and you would break out in cold sweats from time to time. I really hated being on this drug. I didn't feel I had any control of my body when I was on this drug.

This time, things were a little unsettling for me. I had absolutely no idea what was going on. I had no idea what I was going to have to do about work, which was very physical. I had absolutely no idea about anything at all. All I knew was I was alone, I was sick, and I was scared.

I felt I couldn't turn to anyone because, for me, when times get tough you just man up and took care of things. I had no idea how to ask for help or even know who to turn to ask for it. I, as a guy, really hate seeing those words in print let alone using them in real life. I have been a scrapper who rises above all that challenges me. I have a particular distaste for those words because at that time those words were words of weakness. I felt those words showed a weakness in my being a man and being able to take care of myself. I was beginning to question this ability for the first time and it literally frightened me, making me terrified concerning the future.

During this time I went through further testing and I sensed my doctor had no idea what was going on. In the first episode my doctor said she suspected Transverse Myelitis. This is a rare spinal disease that causes the nerve endings in it to deteriorate causing the nerve signals to either misfire or to end completely causing anything from numbness to even paralysis. It is a 1 in 1.3 million chance to get and it rarely shows up twice. I thought I was over it the first time but since it came back so too did the worry of possibly becoming paralyzed.

I believe it was a cold dark Friday evening in November 1998 when I received a call from my doctor explaining some of the tests and her belief that I had Multiple Sclerosis. We hung up the phone and I broke down. I was all alone in a kitchen that evening in the beginnings of winter so it was pitch black outside.

I had no one to call or to talk to and it was in this moment I slowly began to feel my life was over. I now felt a pitch black hole in my soul as dark as the coldest winter night. All that I had known was over. I sat there and sank into a depression for a few hours not knowing what to do or how to fell about any of it.

Me, who had answers for everything, now had nothing.

Nothing.

In my darkest hour I never felt so alone. As if I was in an abyss; all that was good and all future possibilities were being sucked away.

I needed...someone, something, and anything. But I had no one, not a thing and nothing.

That was a hard weekend and a terribly difficult time for me. I didn't really tell anyone what I was told by my doctor; I didn't want to go into why M.S. scared me to my core.

I had moved into a house when I was in 5th grade in a town called Issaquah, Washington. This little sleeper town was an awesome place to grow up. There were plenty of places to travel to, learn and play in. It is nestled in the foothills of the Cascades 15 miles east of Seattle. For being so close to a large city we were in the boondocks.

My backyard was undeveloped park land which lead to a beach on Lake Sammamish. My next door neighbor Dave Scott and I became fast best friends who explored those woods constantly. We would play in the woods that bordered both of our homes. We spent hours and hours in them. We made forts, we built dams along many of the small streams that flowed gently down towards the lake, we explored and through that discovered old telephone wires from decades ago that were hanging from the branches of rather large trees which were at the edge of a sudden drop. We would swing out as far as we could as our own personal "rope swing". That is until it broke with me clinging to that thin wire hoping to return to the safety of the launching area, not crashing face first onto the dozens of small trees lying somewhat flat on the ground. Besides taking the breath out of me it was a great day! These were the times I enjoyed growing up when I got out of the house and explored the world.

At the end of this large undeveloped park was a lake, Lake Sammamish, where we would swim out to the nearest dock as well as spent time on the lake in Dave's boat and other's also. We would also dive for crawdads. Summers were fun while we lived there. I spent as much time outside in those woods or playing various games with all the neighbor kids such as kick the can, capture the flag and hide and seek. It was as much fun as I could expect being a kid.

We lived quite a few miles from town, Issaquah, who had a celebration in the fall every year which celebrated the spawning salmon of all things! It was called Salmon Days. We would jump on our BMX bikes and pedal to town with as much change in our pockets. When we got there we would locate the best vendor bar none every year. Scones. These scones were huge and for .75 cents we got what seemed to be an elephant ear size scone freshly fried in oil with so many toppings it was difficult to choose, so we would sometimes heap a few on each scone. We would then spend the rest of the day either watching the parade or seeing as much of the other venders and events as possible. When we became bored or ran out of money for scones or the other various foodstuffs we would mount up and ride the many miles back home. In a way it felt a bit like the kids in the movie Stand By Me, always an adventure to be had around every corner.

This seemed to be a great place to grow up as a kid and I loved the adventures we would have and the fun they would bring. Those were the fun times during that time period. Looking back I feel it was the time period where I may have actually enjoyed life.

Dave's mother had M.S. and was in a wheelchair. I don't really remember her outside of the home. More or less she stayed indoors the whole time that I lived there. I saw firsthand how this disease affected the human body and hearing those words affected me more than I could let on. To anyone, especially myself. I needed to maintain my composure and be stalwart. I needed to be a man, right?

I saw a bleak future with that possible diagnosis and it weighed down upon me greatly. It affected me on the inside though I obviously couldn't have anyone seeing me falling apart. I was too strong for that. Yet I never felt more helpless. I walked in short steps, almost shuffling to walk anywhere. The house I lived in didn't have but a few stairs; it was an effort to get up and down them. I was fatigued a lot easier by anything I did and my work suffered. I couldn't do half of what I was used to doing.

At the time I worked for a company that ran several apartment complexes which I took care of. There were 225 in all at three locations which I used a rotational schedule to keep them up and well maintained. Before I became ill, I could transport a refrigerator up three flights of stairs by myself. I was strong and able bodied but my weakness due to this illness began to force me to rethink my employment. I didn't have a backup plan so I was forced to resign that November.

The next several months were a blur. I would seemingly feel stronger for about 2 months then I would lose all those gains. My strength came and went like the tide. This went on from November 1998 until June of 1999. Those months were filled with many doctor appointments. One of those appointments, my doctor revealed she had no clue what I had and threw her arms up in defeat. I had bested her knowledge yet she had the ability to tell me this. I have always appreciated her honesty at that time. It must be very difficult for a doctor to vocally admit not knowing what was medically affecting a patient and I hold her in respect for that.

I had another appointment scheduled later that day so I must have sensed a potential ending of our relationship. I went into that appointment with a large manila envelope containing multiple MRI scan results. She asked what I needed help with and I replied, "My spinal cord is swollen." "That can't be," she said, "That's impossible." I said, "I have $20,000 worth of MRI scans proving it is." After the exam I came back to her office and she said in a state of bewilderment that "Yes indeed your spinal cord is swollen" though she asked for 2 weeks to consult some of her colleagues. I agreed.

At the next appointment she was still unable to figure out a course of action. We did more tests. Doctors love tests. I now believe tests are a way for doctors to silently ask for more time while in their heads their inner voice is probably screaming, I HAVE NO IDEA!

It isn't fun to be that patient. As much fun as it is to stump a highly intelligent doctor it really sucks because as a patient all you wish for are answers and solutions in the form of treatment. I, as the patient, wanted things as before. I wanted to be healthy again. I wasn't getting those reassurances from her. Deep inside I was highly displeased with the lack of answers while the outward version of me was laughing and carefree about what was going on with my body. I mean how does someone's spinal cord end up being swollen anyhow? It really is something to experience firsthand.

Always listen to experts. They'll tell you what can't be done, and why. Then do it.

Robert A. Heinlein

Aim 25 Yards Past The Top – (Im)Possible Principle

In my junior year of high school our cross country coach asked us to run down to the city pool, about a mile away from the school. We were going to run hills. Our City pool had a very steep hill on the east side. If anyone has run hills you know that they are hell on earth.

We got to the top the first time and were then instructed to go back down to run another one, this time we were to run to the top and keep going another 25 yards! How many of you have stopped running at the top only to keel over trying to catch your breath! And we were to run another 25 yards?? I hurt so badly. I had to dig deep in order to not keel over and puke my guts out.

After practicing this new skill over the coming month we finally were able to see it in action at our first meet. I learned something interesting that race. I totally blew by 4 or 5 competing runners in those 25 yards. I also never saw them again. What was most intriguing to me was in that 25 yards I had caught my breath and I had regained my strength without ever slowing down!! With the right plan that was different than any other cross country team and the mindset to work harder than everyone else one can accomplish a lot more than usual.

I had not only physically beaten these other runners but I had beaten them psychologically. I defeated them physically and therefore I beat them mentally. I learned a new skill set and I worked harder than the other person. I was willing to do more than him when it came to life and I was therefore willing to work harder to learn to walk again.

I was willing to put in the work. Period.

There will be obstacles
There will be doubters
There will be mistakes
But with hard work
There are no limits

Life Will Slow You Down, Sometimes With Paralysis

In June of 1999 I was forced to move yet again due to my roommate getting married. I literally moved a half mile up the road. I had to say goodbye to the best bachelor pad I've ever lived. This new place was a good place for me to move as it was one level and only had two small half steps to enter it. That was a Monday. On Friday I began to notice my legs becoming weaker and weaker. I began to walk all jerky and unsure of each step. I scheduled another MRI for that Monday morning. I needed a friend to pick me up and drive me since my legs had really deteriorated fast over the weekend.

I stumbled into her car but by the time we got to the clinic for the MRI I needed a hospital type wheelchair to make it into the room for the scan. Upon completion of the MRI, I went to sit up and I could not move my legs. I sat there perplexed for a couple seconds. I tried again. Nope. I couldn't move my legs now.

Great.

Even better than that was I also discovered I had urinated on myself during the MRI. I was now paralyzed from the chest down so I couldn't feel the need to use the bathroom nor that I wet myself. I would have to say that was rather embarrassing but that is an understatement. I was kind of freaking out inside that I couldn't feel or move anything from the chest down. There was nothing to do but have the tech lady call my doctor who told me to go to the hospital to check in and she would meet me there to run tests and find out what was going on. Luckily I was in a clinic in the corner of the same lot as the hospital so I just pushed myself in the wheelchair to the entrance and checked myself in.

In a way, I remember feeling glad to have other people taking care of me. I kind of liked not having to worry about those little things like food shopping, laundry, or cleaning up. I was in the ICU at first and while I know it was a hospital I had friends over for movie parties until at least 1:30 in the morning several times. I lived it up as a Very Important Guest of this hospital. It was the end of June, the 22nd to be exact.

I was in serious, delusional denial. Or I had a handle on the situation that no one could figure out. I was calm. I was laughing, and having a blast, forgetting that I was paralyzed from the chest down. I mean who does that? Denial is powerful. Or was I a visionary.

As the 4th of July was coming soon I had a friend bring a goody bag in full of fireworks. Of course I couldn't light many, fine, none of them but I found a certain satisfaction in throwing the pop-its at my

44

nurses. I would wait till they were checking my blood pressure and listening to my heart and to me breathe when I would toss one behind them freaking them out. Yes, I was that kind of patient but it was stress relief for me. I have to say that this was all fun and games until one day I got a Godzilla nurse, you know the ones who are like 6 feet tall and at least 5 feet wide and scary in their demeanor. Yea, that one. She was intimidating to say the least. She came in the first, and only, time to say that she needed to check my 'Hiney.' She actually said hiney. I asked what for and she said for bedsores. Well, I had only been in there some 4 days is all so I informed her there will be no hiney looking here. And I also said I have pop its and was prepared to use them! Well, she didn't take to kindly to this and I obligingly did not toss one in her direction. I was aware enough of my personal safety in the hands of one who could make or break my experience there!

I was moved to the rehab floor soon after this to begin the recovery process. In those first few days I was able to get back up after the drugs had lessened the swelling of my spinal cord and stand. With my weaker left leg in a blow up brace it allowed me to walk up and down the length of the parallel bars building up strength. I would also be stretched and worked on in other ways to help invigorate my legs.

I began to have muscle contractions and spasms in my legs and lower torso the previous October, Halloween to be exact. If you have

45

never experienced involuntary spasms, it was nearly a minute of extremely severe nerve pain akin to being on fire. I don't remember how many or how often they were up until that point but they weren't too common at the time. However, I began to have many in the hospital and especially in rehab. I remember once when I had one on the raised mat in rehab and my whole body arched in the air with only my feet and shoulder blades touching the mat and I groaned and grunted although I just wanted to scream out loud. It was extreme and it was severe, intense pain. Nothing I said to the doctor there got me any relief either. I'm not sure if it was my lack of describing how intensely painful it was or his lack of truly caring but it was a difficult time because of that. It may have been my willingness to suck up a bunch of pain in order to not be seen as a whiner. Again, my manliness stood in the way I'm sure.

I was in the hospital for a bit longer than 8 days for this one; I was in there for 6 weeks and, it at times, seemed to go on forever. With physical therapy daily and therefore pain daily it made those days so much longer than I can ever describe. I made friends with other patients. I especially remember one older gentleman who had had a stroke. He found himself on the floor unable to use one side of his body and had to pull himself to a phone to call for help. This took him quite a long time to do and when I met him it was in rehab so he could gain strength and movement on that one side. He had a gruff exterior that was behind some of the things he would say.

He was pretty down about life obviously and I don't remember him receiving many visitors if any at all. We became fast friends. I would go over to his room, which was right next to mine and talk. He was a good guy who I am sure was quite fearful of a life full of physical issues that might cause him to need to reach out to others for help. It is a very hard thing for an otherwise healthy individual to have to learn. Especially if you have not needed that help from others in your life?

Once I was released to go home I set up home health again and began having physical therapists come over and continue the work to get me walking under my own power again. I spent several months with these home health physical therapists coming over twice a week to help me use a walker to gain strength in my legs. I got up to about 100 yards in the walker by walking out my house down the lane to the mailboxes. I began to think that maybe this strange scary episode would be over soon. Boy was I wrong.

Difficult doesn't mean impossible it simply means you have to work hard.

Let's See What Else Will Happen

This time period is a little murky looking back but in December of 1999 my legs went paralyzed again from the chest down over a couple days. I found myself heading to the E.R. again and found myself once again in the hospital. This time the emergency room doctor was ready to send me home. He was, quite frankly, the biggest jerk doctor I had ever met up to that time. He seemed to challenge my even being in the emergency room. He told me to go home and call my doctor. I told him I wasn't leaving until he talked to my doctor. We had a stare down, which I won. He put me in a back room and came back several hours later. He asked me if I had a ride home. I told him I wasn't leaving until I talked to my doctor. Again, we stared each other down and I won again. He left and soon my doctor showed up did a small assessment and said yup, I'll admit you to the hospital for treatment. Why did it seem like I had to convince everybody that I was bad off and needed help? Don't they understand how difficult it is to even ask for help?

A couple days after that I found that my left arm stopped working from the shoulder down. I could hardly lift it. I definitely couldn't move it from the elbow or move a single finger or even make a fist. While I was obviously a bit overwhelmed the biggest shock came a day or two later when I went in for a spinal tap. I was on the table face down so they could insert the needle into my back to retrieve the fluid they needed to be able to tell what was happening to me and if there were any anomalies in the fluid.

One thing you need to get about me is I like messing with doctors. I love cracking jokes and really just messing with them. So, as usual I went to crack a funny on the doctors performing the procedure and as I went to say something my ears were shocked by what they heard. You've heard a baby coo and blabber right?

Yes, that's what I heard coming from my mouth, while what I heard inside my head was the funniest thing they never heard. I was shocked. I was alarmed. I attempted to say something else, and the same sound was heard. It freaked me out so bad, I was now more scared than I have ever been.

As I left the procedure room and went back to my room I let the doctor's know that something else was wrong. I had another MRI that showed that my spinal cord had a lesion on it in the neck area. This affected my speech and left me quite literally speechless!

What was especially weird was around 6 p.m. that evening I was able to form words that made sense and I felt obvious relief at the progress in such a short amount of time. I awoke the next morning and the same exact thing happened. I went to speak and gobbledygook came out. By this time I was so distressed about this and the effects upon my speech. I cherish speech. I am expert at talking, ask anyone who has met me. I always have something to say and I will always say it. It is my tool. It was now a broken tool and neither I nor the doctors (who are advertised as all wise) knew what happened to it or how to get it back. I was so distressed that when my friend Paul Fetzer came that evening to visit me (he's like my adopted dad) I broke down and asked what was going on. I was lacking the thing that makes things make sense to me, knowledge. I needed to know what was going on in order to process it and understand it.

The next day nothing further occurred I cautiously felt I was hopefully able to move on. The only problem that remained was a voice that had some issues. My voice sounded much higher pitched and I struggled to form words to speak. In fact it was tiring. I had to figure out the quickest way to say what needed to be said in the fewest amount of words anytime I needed to speak. Otherwise, my words would become slurred and I would tire easily.

I was then directed to a speech therapist. When I rolled into her office and she said that because I am speaking I should just keep on speaking more. I sat there in disbelief that this is what a trained speech therapist is telling me to do. Go and speak more. Wow, I thought, my insurance company is going to be paying a hell of a lot of money for me to speak more! Of course, my friends hate me ever since because I talk...a lot!

My left arm was still paralyzed with no movement or sense of feeling. I had a flaccid arm from the shoulder down. Well, two weeks into having no use of it, on a Sunday late in the evening, I was lying there in bed watching television when my left pinky twitched! I was shocked and excited that it had decided to show some life. The next morning I excitedly told the physical therapist what had happened the night before and he immediately began to ask me to move it and to do this and that until I couldn't move it anymore, which didn't take long. I regretted telling him that it twitched. Twice a day he did these exercises on it until it was dead. That length of time increased gradually each day but by the end of each day it returned to uselessness until a few weeks into this routine I had gained back all I was going to gain back. I still had some residual numbness which increased from the shoulder to the fingers, the fingers being number than the rest of the arm, and it still is today but I am used to it and it does not impede me.

Physical therapy was tough. My legs were paralyzed, my left arm stayed paralyzed for 2 weeks and my speech was, with effort, coming back. I was a pile of conundrums. I had one good arm. They tried to get me to use it through real world activities like cooking. They have a working kitchen to teach life skills so I made brownies! They were, of course, the best brownies I have ever tasted! I would participate in fine motor skill challenges such as putting slick metal posts into a board with holes in it. They were tough to pick up with my still recovering fingers that felt little and were very dry so they weren't very easy to grasp. It was frustrating to do something so easy so poorly. I would be timed. I am competitive by nature so I naturally attempt to push the limits. I was really bothered when the outcome didn't match my vision.

After 6 weeks in the hospital, I was finally released to go home. It was a happy time but also one of confusion. I and my cadre of professionals still didn't know what was causing all these issues in my spinal cord. No one had a clue and it left me in the dark. What do I do next? Who do I see about it? Where were answers hiding? I was paralyzed chest down and no doctor would tell me I would walk again. I would say it but they would neither acknowledge what I said or they would change the subject. No one believed I would walk again. Yet, I knew deep down in places I couldn't explain that I would indeed walk again. I just needed to research and find the right treatment that could help me do that.

For the next several years I would seek out knowledge and doctors who might know what was going on. Not a single doctor enjoyed appointments with me asking what was going on and how do I heal from it. Apparently, I got enough of a reputation that I couldn't find another doctor to take my case. I was stuck and stuck doesn't get you answers.

The only way to discover the limits of the possible is to go beyond them into the impossible.

Arthur C. Clarke

And Then Life Went To Hell

The next few years were a blur of doctors mixed with ebb and flow of physical improvement and regression. I would get to a high point of standing and, only once, I was able to take a few steps while holding on to a rail. I could never really get past that point. In the spring of 2003, I noticed a red blotch on my left leg. It looked like a sort of birthmark looking blob shape that was deep red in color. I went to a dermatologist and she didn't really know what it was so she referred me to a doctor at the University of Utah by the name of Doctor Zone. I loved his name, 'I'm in the zone" became a silent little mantra of mine. He took one look at my leg and said I had Lupus, but that he would take a biopsy to confirm.

Luckily I had learned what that was during my own research so it wasn't the biggest shock in the world. I had Lupus. What does a guy do with this though? How is it treated? Does it affect my long term survival? I had a lot of questions but in the end it is a disease that affects the muscles, joints, organs and many other symptoms like heat sensitivity, sun sensitivity and extreme exhaustion. This occurs mostly in women, in fact 90% of Lupus patients are women. Does that mean I am getting in touch with my feminine side? I have a woman's disease? Really? Wow, blow to my manhood complete.

I took this news in stride. It meant that we were getting closer the overall answers. I cannot express the significance to me at the time. I find humans need progression to have the sense that things are going somewhere rather than feeling stagnant. Hope started trickling into my soul.

October of 2003 I flew to LA for my best friend's wedding. It was a whirlwind couple of days and I remember having a blast and really enjoying the whole experience. It was on a wedding yacht that had three stories, lots of windows, and it toured around Newport Harbor for the afternoon. It was a really beautiful day to commemorate my friend's wonderful occasion. Of course, being the best man allowed me to converse with all the beautiful bridesmaids and I applied my speech therapists counsel well! All were enchanted by the wondrous environment. Positive thoughts permeated my mind all weekend.

I do not remember anything after leaving my friend's wedding celebration until I was picked up from the floor of my bedroom semi-conscious. It could have been days or weeks; I was found on my bedroom floor by a friend who freaked out and called our mutual friend Paul Fetzer.

My friend Paul Fetzer's face was in mine. I was prostrate and somewhat dismayed at being interrupted and yelled at. Paul was loudly talking, completely in my face trying to stir me awake. I was somewhat obstinate in my replies telling him to leave me alone. I was very put out by his yelling.

The next thing I remember is being in the back of an ambulance heading down my lane. I next remember feeling like I needed to pick my nose because there was something large, soft and annoying in my nostril. An Asian woman in a smock tried to get me to not pick at it since it turned out to be a blood clot. Apparently they performed some procedure and I needed to leave it be.

I do not remember much during this time, I have no idea how long I was in the hospital. It is a period of time where time and space do not meet up and even begin to make sense to me. I still have no recollection and many unanswered questions concerning this time period and would like to know all that occurred at some point.

What I do know is this. They found 36 lesions in my brain. I found out some years later that the doctor told everyone that I would die that night. If I woke up I would be a vegetable for the rest of my life. I also found out some years later that my brothers' then wife was there and overheard my mother tell the doctors to not keep me on life support. I had no real contact with her yet she flew down from Seattle requesting the doctors let me die? Who does that? Request that their son is allowed to pass away. I still don't have the words since hearing that this occurred. Apparently, things were pretty dire!

I next remember being on a cold metal table and being asked to lay flat on my back with my head turned to I believe the left side and I was not to move it at all. It was extremely hot. I was receiving an angiogram. I was on this table thinking to myself, "why am I getting something done that is only for old people with heart problems." I couldn't comprehend what the heck I was doing there nor did I have the presence of mind to say anything or to protest this procedure.

It was extremely hot and I was sweating and extraordinarily uncomfortable lying there. It seemed to go on forever until it was done. I was on a stretcher going out a door that took me onto the street that separated the main hospital and a large stale looking building where apparently tests and procedures were performed.

I can only assume later that day a woman entered my room. She sat down and began to talk about my heart and something about a hole and a surgery. You'll have to put yourself in my shoes for a minute to get proper perspective on what was going through my mind at this moment. I had picked up racing a hand cycle a couple years before and had just won a marathon the month before. So I was in pretty decent shape as far as my cardio and blood pressure. I countered what she was saying and couldn't and probably wouldn't let any of this sink in. I had a hole in my heart and it was rather large as these things go.

I was told it was very common and in fact she had just operated upon her own 11 year old son. She left my room and I was left to ponder this news alone. I needed heart surgery to close a hole in my heart.

While I am not afraid of surgery, I seemed to have a hard time believing I needed heart surgery. There is a more serious connotation with this kind of surgery and it was hitting me rather hard. How does a man who just won a marathon on a hand bike for paraplegics come to need heart surgery? I was dumbfounded, I had no idea who to even turn to. It turns out that when they scanned me when I arrived at the hospital and was found to have all those 36 lesions in my brain. My brother told me much later that is where they stopped counting there were so many in there. But looking back it is important to notice that they found something up there and I could rest assured that it had been confirmed that I indeed had a brain.

Needless to say, my thinking wasn't really firing on all cylinders. There was a lot I couldn't grasp and there was even more I couldn't find the words to understand nor could I formulate an articulate question and lacked the ability to talk to someone about it. I was extremely frustrated and couldn't express it. That is why the revelation that I needed heart surgery to close a hole was very other worldly to me.

A few days later, the date was set for the surgery. Halloween. Yes, I was to have heart surgery on Halloween to fix my broken heart. A trick or treat? I thought it was rather appropriate.

The day before surgery my brother Todd showed up with his wife and kid. I hadn't seen him since at least his wedding reception at our house in Issaquah some 8 or nine years before. We didn't keep in touch up until that time so I was rather surprised at this. I only remember that at the time the Red Cross evacuated him out of South Korea where he was stationed in the Army. I only learned some years later that a Soldier only gets out of there if someone in the family is dying. Since my doctor believed I was dying, that gave him his get out of jail free card.

The next day I had to mark my body with a sharpie pen so that the surgeon wouldn't make a mistake about which leg they were going to insert the catheter in to perform the surgery. This is inserted up the carotid artery and push it up to my heart to insert a device made out of titanium or some alloy that would enter the hole and expand on either side of the hole in my heart and then clamp over the heart tissue, sealing the hole. I wouldn't even have a scar to brag about and show the women. I was really disappointed by this news.

I awoke with a nasty metallic taste in my mouth. Kind of like some laser surgery was performed in my mouth. It was nasty and my teeth felt weird and out of place. I really hated waking up to that. The bed I was in was placed in an area for partial recovery and my friend Paul was there to greet me and to accompany me. I only remember him looking at the machines I was attached to monitoring my blood pressure and heart rate and him asking me if I could purposely lower my heart rate. Somehow it lowered down to 50 within a few minutes.

He was impressed and it was also kind of fun to toy with things like that.

After some time in this area I was wheeled to what I thought would be my old room. I was brought to a corner room that was on the corner of two hallways, so an outside corner room if you will. It felt claustrophobic to me and I asked when we were going back to my room. I was told this is my new room. I balked at this. I wanted familiarity, no, I needed familiarity. I really needed this more than I could comprehend at the time. And it is weird that I stood up for this request making it into a demand. I freaked out. I went wacko, I became unhinged enough to unnerve them. To the point of getting the intern there to tell me that this was my room and I am to stay there until I remembered which hospital I was in, what room I was in and what day it was, he was also firm that I get a full night of sleep as well. He was seriously firm on this and it wasn't a request but a very stern, 'you are doing this no matter how you feel about it' kind of manner. I was pretty pissed off to say the least because I told him ALL HOSPITALS ARE THE SAME INSIDE! I was firm with that statement knowing full well I had no clue. I did not know what hospital I was in. I did not know what day it was. I had no clue about anything except I was in one and I just had heart surgery!

He left and I was left to figure those things out somehow. I was so frustrated and upset and really truly discombobulated.

My brother and his family came to visit me post-op. I have no recollection. It may be due to what my brother related to me years later. His observation was I had an 11 second memory capacity and could not conceive of anything outside of the room door. I would ask him when I was going back to my hospital room. He would reply I was in my hospital room. I would then ask what was outside the room door, being told it was the rest of the hospital. This repeated for about 45 minutes. The aide came back at this time to ask if I remember which hospital I was in and I replied with the name of a hospital six miles away.

Very soon thereafter a small handful of friends came to the hospital to visit and I quickly tried to hatch a plan of escape. I tried to convince Daniel and Marianne, friends of mine who were dating, to unlock the wheels of my bed and to push me out the door to the elevator just the opposing side of the door to the room I was in. It was maybe 25-30 feet to freedom as I had formulated in my mind. They were of course leery of this line of thought from me and were concerned about my plan. They tried to encourage me to stay and recuperate. But in my mind this was the perfect plan and I couldn't understand why they would not help me out. An understandable position right?

They soon left after a pretty good visit despite my psycho exit plan. Once they left I was on my own to try and figure out the list of things I needed to remember. Looking back I'm sure they truly thought I had lost it. And looking back I had. I really did have a mental breakdown that night.

My mind, which was broken, overloaded on reality and it literally broke. I began to think of the preceding 8 days that I figured I was in the hospital and I was rather shocked to discover that I had not slept more than a wink or two in those 8 days. See, I was on many drugs for pain, muscle spasms, nerve calming medicine and many others totaling about 50 pills a day. Some were narcotic in nature and rendered me just a little messed up. I was on oxycodone, OxyContin, 50 mcg fentanyl patches, morphine, Ambien, and many others.

I began to slowly realize that I was taken off all these drugs when I was brought in to the hospital roughly 8 days previous and because I was taken off all these drugs at once I had not slept at all during this time. I had been awake for 8 days straight and I had had surgery. The anesthesia I was given for this surgery was the catalyst in my mental breakdown. To be deprived of sleep for so long due to going cold turkey off so many medicines forced me over the edge and my mind broke.

It became apparent that I needed to sleep, reset my mind and to get out of the hospital. Now, my memory is not all too clear, I believe either that night or the next, I really am not sure, but I got 6 hours of poor sleep and not in a row. I remember feeling as though I had awoken to a new day and a new beginning. I really felt great. I called the intern in and told him that I know who I am and that I had slept that night and I felt I needed to be released back to my own home to begin the healing process in surroundings that I felt would be more conducive to that, while I have no idea which hospital I am in I was going to be leaving that day and that whether he would advise that or not, I was leaving and that he should go call the doctor, who was on vacation, that I would be leaving today with or without his permission. He came back an hour and a half later to acknowledge that I would be discharged shortly.

I arrived home to an extraordinarily clean home, such a one I have never known. I mean this was cleaner than when I moved in. It felt sterile and almost too clean. But it was nice not to be in a hospital. The only problem I ran into was my inability to remember my passwords to my computer. Try as I might I couldn't remember them. It took me almost two weeks before I did and it was frustrating to me during this time. I felt extraordinarily helpless and alone and absolutely not sure what to do.

My brain had been overloaded and it broke down. My mind was my greatest asset. In college I had almost a photographic memory and could remember things in books to the smallest degree. If a classmate asked where I found something I could tell them which of a hundred books on the table it was, which page, whether it was the right or left column, which paragraph, and which line it was found. I prided myself on remembering many things as I needed them to be recalled and I lost this ability. It was my greatest asset. When I lost my voice I really felt my life was over because I needed the ability to communicate with others. I felt it was what connected me with others and validated me in some way and to lose that seemed to automatically cut me off from others. Losing my memory was worse by far.

This was a totally different ballgame now. I had truly reset my brain and no one knew what the consequences were. I felt a loneliness I had never known. I was literally a shell of my former self and I knew it. I was also dealing with the fact that I had been cut off cold turkey from 4 narcotics that my body was addicted to. At the time, I had no idea of these things. I knew that my personality changed and I would be in conversations with others and jokes would be cracked and everyone would be laughing except me. Yet inside my mind I was asking myself why I wasn't laughing. I could not connect the reasons why. I couldn't relate to people for some time after the removal of these narcotics. My body was freaking out. It went into shock after the removal of the medicines in addition to the 4 narcotics I was on. It was going through withdrawals and I didn't know it. Hell, I'm not sure my doctor knew what he did. I could have and probably should have died from the shock of going cold turkey off these narcotics. I do not know how I survived.

This period was hard on my mind. It took months for my personality to begin showing again. For those many months I literally was a zombie of sorts, I couldn't laugh or get into it with others. I comprehend what addicts suffer through and it took several months in which I slowly melted this wall or shell until I could reemerge the person I am. I have a lot of respect for those who have had to enter drug rehab. I can't imagine going through drug rehab through your own volition to experience all that physical adjustment and mental pain.

After I got home and was able to finally access my computer, I emailed my friend Lee, she was going to medical school when I met her, and was now a doctor. I thought she was in New York doing residency and I emailed her about the Lupus and the stroke. She emailed me back and was surprised about the Lupus part. The next day she emailed me again to report that she was at the National Institutes of Health in Bethesda, Maryland. She went and talked with the rheumatology department and they said they'd be interested in receiving my records and would look at them but could not promise me anything but that they would at least look.

I was stoked about this and over the next couple months was able to gain access to all of my records and had them sent to this doctor at the NIH in Bethesda, Maryland. Roughly two months later or so, in the middle of January, I was at lunch with a friend, Gary, who mentioned that if I ever needed to fly anywhere to let him know as he had airplane vouchers to use. Well, as soon as I got home from this lunch I received a call from a heavily accented man who identified himself as being from NIH and after some small talk asked if I wanted to come out for a visit and be seen by him. I said I'd fly out tomorrow if I needed. He offered the week after that Sunday for the trip and I agreed. The date saving my life and changing it forever was set.

I called Gary up after we hung up and asked if that offer of the voucher was still good, he replied yes it was and he set me up with the flight. I was pretty happy about this and for some reason felt that this was exactly the thing I needed to gain some progress towards discovering exactly what was wrong with my body and to figure out how to fix it. I was elated and I knew this was a pivotal moment in my life. It burned within me that this was a major opportunity.

What was even better is I had a friend, Emily, who lived in DC now and she agreed to pick me up from the airport and take me to the NIH. As we sat in the waiting area, we learned about the Super Bowl and Janet Jackson's booby problem. I will remember that date eternally because I was happy that I didn't have to witness her "malfunction."

Monday morning I met with the docs for the first time. There was Illei who was Hungarian, an Indian woman and a woman from the Deep South, all doctors of various specialties. I literally had to pause a minute between each one to focus on their accent as each of them were very deep and rich. It was the hardest conversation I think I have ever had. Basically they were going to test me in some areas and get some blood samples and discuss what the potential diseases were and try to diagnose me. I was ecstatic and very happy about this development.

Well, on Wednesday night all three came into my room, I remember it was 6 that night; they told me that they all believed I had Transverse Myelitis and Lupus. Since I had researched both and was very familiar with them I nodded and said so what's next? I believe that they were expecting me to mourn or something, feel sadness or to breakdown and cry because they just stood there a little taken back by my direct response. I had been living with this thing for so long not much could shock or surprise me, I merely wanted to move on and get crackalackin on treating it.

The reply from Illei Gabor was they would recommend a 6 month course of chemotherapy. I asked frequency and they said monthly. I asked if I was to start there or when I got home and how to get the doctors there to agree to this course of action. They said I could start there. I wanted this as it would take a month for my doctors to pull their collective heads out. So it was set up for me to start there. My friend Emily who picked me up from the airport was able to show me around DC and Arlington National Cemetery. Might as well make a vacation out of the trip.

Many times we are our worst enemy. If we could learn to conquer ourselves, then we will have a much easier time overcoming the obstacles that are in front of us.

Stephen Labossiere

Wrecks Happen But So Do The Signs – (Im)Possible Principle

I broke my left leg into chicken nugget pieces when I crashed my hand cycle in a 10 k race for failing to make a turn properly at 25 miles an hour. Okay, I made the turn properly but I sort of ran into a concrete median that just jumped out in front of me and since my legs are out in front on a hand bike my left leg took the brunt of the force of my body and bike coming to a sudden stop at that speed. I apparently flipped one and a half times around to land on my left side according to the cop/paramedic observing from the corner. I shattered my left tibia and fibia and dented my tibia plateau (the top of the tibia bone) 5 millimeters and cracked my helmet in half.

Let's put it this way, I didn't have time to get my swear out!

All week I had feelings that I shouldn't do the race. The night before my sunglasses broke and I spent time finding super glue at the store when I should have been at home resting. There were other signs, I ignored them all and I ended up shattering my leg. I required surgery, 4 metal plates, 14 screws and some fake bone. It has caused me problems ever since that could have been avoided had I listened to those signs. My left ankle and knee are a bother every single day ever since but I learned a valuable lesson to always trust your gut, no matter what.

It's okay to change your plans; Life doesn't usually conform to your ideals and visions. If you're to grow you will have to learn to adapt and change your plans for a better path even though it won't look like it at first. Trust your gut and all will reveal itself to you.

The more obstacles I overcome the stronger I become.

Gracie Alvarez

Chemo And The Finish Line

The next few months grew into a routine of a monthly chemo where I would go in to the hospital/clinic and receive my dose. After a few treatments I felt the same and asked the nurse that if I was supposed to feel tired and worn out and all the usual chemo questions. I was only asking because I felt great. It was a weird reaction and one that I wasn't really prepared for. I felt I needed to add to the story and enter a marathon. I emailed Ogden Marathon and they cleared me to enter. I had roughly 4 weeks to get race ready. So I got started by riding every day. The day of the race came and my friend Paul Philips agreed to go up with me and even offered up his aunt's couch since she lived close to the race start. We drove the race course that night as was my custom to help me visualize my race.

Once we got to her place to sleep I couldn't. One of the side effects of chemo for me was an exaggerated insomnia. I had been averaging 1-2 hours' sleep for the previous several months and this was no exception. I got a whole hour and a bit of sleep. The race start temperature was below freezing, 55 gal barrels of fire were interspersed and I sat next to one trying to keep warm.

The start was fast and lightly downhill....for 6 miles before it turned a sharp right and went to a small town where it turned left to begin the course around the reservoir to the end of it where it met the top of the canyon we had to go down. I was out front at this time wondering where everyone was but not wanting to turn back to look as it might upset my mojo. I just kept motoring. It was this course where I discovered why one would want to win a race, police escort!

I had a highway patrol with lights on 20-30 yards in front of me bleeping his siren to announce someone was coming. I was coming and I loved this, it was awesome!

Once we had started the race about 10 minutes into it, it began to downpour, in fact the cloud coming over the mountain was dark, black, and angry looking. I knew this was going to open up and dump so it motivated me to hurry up. I got to the top of the canyon and by this time it was dumping fast, dense big drops were hitting all around me. I got up to 40 mph going down the canyon and near the bottom I saw 2 bicycle cops who were to take over from the patrol car and escort me along the bike path to town and Main Street where it led to the finish line. I blew by the first cop and the second was up on his feet ahead of me constantly looking back. Once we made it to Main Street, I was talking to him and Chemotherapy came up and how my next treatment, my 5th, was the following week. He was pretty amazed. I finished in first place. I was frozen and soaking wet but pretty excited that I had finished, let alone won a 26.2 mile race while undergoing chemotherapy. I knew it was a great story to tell my grandkids someday!

The next few months were fairly uneventful as I went to chemo monthly and tried to think good things in regards to this treatment staying the effects of this disease. I finished in July and just kept living day to day with the hope that the chemo would keep me in a good place.

In the middle of October 2004 the worst case scenario occurred. The right side of my body became paralyzed. Literally, right down the center of my body. My right arm and right leg were paralyzed. It certainly made pushing a wheelchair rather difficult. Talk about going in circles.

I was devastated that I only received 9 months of peace with this treatment. I was sure it would give me more than that and I was angry about it. Now what was I going to do? I can push a wheelchair in some pretty sweet circles and that got me nowhere. I was really at wits end with this. I finally had received a diagnosis after 6 years of searching and going through unimaginable effects on my body and mind only to go paralyzed. Again.

I was to a point of despair, and I don't do despair.

I called the NIH and Dr. Gabor to report that I had a relapse of symptoms and what can we do about it. We made arrangements to fly out there for a week of screening for a study. They had told me back in February there was a high risk study if this chemotherapy treatment failed to work.

One of my best friends, Marc Western, gave me a ticket to Maryland and I went out for a week of screening for this study. I was pretty upbeat and hopeful that this was a very real possibility for me. After about 4 or 5 days they came to me to discuss the study and my involvement in it. The doctors and researcher there don't really come out and ask if you want to be in the study. He, in a sense, said that I am a great candidate for this study, if I would stay. Of course my answer would be hell yea. So, I asked if they wanted me to stay, they acknowledged that they would. I changed my flight and stayed. That is how I came to be included in their study. It felt strange but I was a great candidate for their experiment!

The study involved a stem cell transplant extracted from my own cells in the hopes that they could cure my Lupus. It was revolutionary and bold. Using my own body to heal itself of an incurable autoimmune disease. I was all in.

But by God sometimes you have to be able to think about the unthinkable.

Ursula K. LeGuin

It Wasn't From My Rib, But Close Enough (A New Life Is Born)

What are stem cells and what is the controversy surrounding them? Stem cells came on the public horizon around 2000 or 2001 in a big way. Touted for their apparent healing potential in treating a variety of diseases and possibly even spinal cord injuries. The buzz was very loud and yet full of hope. They were extremely controversial due to then current technology for two types discussed. The first were adult donor cells and the second was embryonic stem cells. The latter source proved to be an issue with the public and they were decried on a massive scale based on ethical grounds. The public seemed to decry stem cells as a whole believing it unethical and inhumane to produce an embryo only to destroy it to collect the stem cells. I won't get into the argument here but there is more to this than meets the eye. I believe it is up to everyone to formulate their own opinion based upon solid fact and not conjecture and half-truths.

The following information I copied directly off the National Institutes of Health's own website so as to not include my interpretation. It is great information and is advancing all the time so please visit nih.gov for your own education and edification.

75

Stem cells have the remarkable potential to develop into many different cell types in the body during early life and growth. In addition, in many tissues they serve as a sort of internal repair system, dividing essentially without limit to replenish other cells as long as the person or animal is still alive. When a stem cell divides, each new cell has the potential either to remain a stem cell or become another type of cell with a more specialized function, such as a muscle cell, a red blood cell, or a brain cell.

Stem cells are distinguished from other cell types by two important characteristics. First, they are unspecialized cells capable of renewing themselves through cell division, sometimes after long periods of inactivity. Second, under certain physiologic or experimental conditions, they can be induced to become tissue- or organ-specific cells with special functions. In some organs, such as the gut and bone marrow, stem cells regularly divide to repair and replace worn out or damaged tissues. In other organs, however, such as the pancreas and the heart, stem cells only divide under special conditions.

Given their unique regenerative abilities, stem cells offer new potentials for treating diseases such as diabetes, and heart disease. However, much work remains to be done in the laboratory and the clinic to understand how to use these cells for cell-based therapies to treat disease, which is also referred to as regenerative or reparative medicine.

Laboratory studies of stem cells enable scientists to learn about the cells' essential properties and what makes them different from specialized cell types. Scientists are already using stem cells in the laboratory to screen new drugs and to develop model systems to study normal growth and identify the causes of birth defects.

Research on stem cells continues to advance knowledge about how an organism develops from a single cell and how healthy cells replace damaged cells in adult organisms. Stem cell research is one of the most fascinating areas of contemporary biology, but, as with many expanding fields of scientific inquiry, research on stem cells raises scientific questions as rapidly as it generates new discoveries.

Stem cells differ from other kinds of cells in the body. All stem cells—regardless of their source—have three general properties: they are capable of dividing and renewing themselves for long periods; they are unspecialized; and they can give rise to specialized cell types.

Stem cells are capable of dividing and renewing themselves for long periods. *Unlike muscle cells, blood cells, or nerve cells—which do not normally replicate themselves—stem cells may replicate many times, or proliferate. A starting population of stem cells that proliferates for many months in the laboratory can yield millions of cells. If the resulting cells continue to be unspecialized, like the parent stem cells, the cells are said to be capable of long term self-renewal.*

There is a vast amount of information available on the National Institutes of Health's website and other places. There is a massive amount of research taking place so please do your research if you are unsure of how you feel about this issue and inform yourself. Don't believe everything you hear. This topic is a hot one for a reason and it will be necessary to know for yourself how you feel about it. Don't take my word for it. For my stem cell transplant my own stem cells were to be used. These incredibly creative researchers figured out how my own body can be used to heal itself. It is science fiction become science fact.

The purpose of the stem cell transplant was to eradicate the lymphocytes and monocytes in my immune system that were bad. Those two cell types are the reason I have Lupus. These two cells attack the bad bacteria and viruses in an otherwise healthy person. In Lupus they do not stop at just the bad, they cannot differentiate and attack the good and the bad without stopping. For me the results are Lupus. For others it is Multiple Sclerosis. Everyone is different but a part of the reason for me were those two cells.

As part of the study, I went through very thorough testing. I was constantly poked and prodded. I had bone marrow biopsies, I had lymph node biopsies. Both of these required a rather large needle to be placed in different locations to extract different materials that would provide the necessary base readings in order to track the progress of the stem cell transplant. The bone marrow biopsy required them to dig through my buttock to dig into the bone of my pelvis. Once the fragment of bone was taken out, a syringe was placed in the opening and the marrow was extracted by pulling the plunger out. Although I was paralyzed, I could feel the vacuum being created through the sucking power of the syringe. It was extremely uncomfortable and quite painful. I can't imagine how that would feel if I could feel my legs!

The lymph nodes were taken from my inner thighs, arm pit and neck with a 5 inch needle. The thigh and arm pits were okay to deal with but the neck? Try placing a sharp needle just under your tongue and press upwards. This is how bad the needle felt except it was inserted into my neck. These along with many MRI's, PET scans and CAT scans and a few x-rays to cover anything else they missed. I was feeling like a CIA torture victim by the end of each and every day!

Once all these tests were carried out I was given 3 different chemotherapies over 5 days. I was a little taken aback by the lack of any real negative symptoms the first time I did chemotherapy the year before. This time I was not let off the hook. I felt the full fury of its side effects this time around.

It soon became difficult to even lift my head from the pillow. I would become out of breath if I did just that. It was all I could do to sit up. Swinging my legs over the edge of the bed was near impossible for me. If I needed to do that I needed to be fully committed for it exhausted me terribly.

Once we finished the chemotherapy sessions we waited three days to begin the infusion.

January 4th 2005, the day that was to change my life completely. The infusion was to last maybe 20 minutes. You would think I might stay alert for that pivotal day but no. I fell asleep due to my extreme, tortured exhaustion. The day that would alter the rest of my life and I fell asleep before the infusion of my own stem cells finished.

When we infused my own stem cells back into me it did a couple things. One, the body said hey, I don't have any of these guys and two, it used these stem cells as templates to resupply my immune system with lymphocytes and monocytes to do their job to attack the bad guys. Only this time...they worked properly.

Think of rebooting a computer. It is, in a manner of speaking, quite similar to that process. We rebooted my body's ability to work properly. In fact, the first thing I felt about 10 days after the infusion was either a lack of fatigue or I felt a level of energy I hadn't felt in seven years.

That realization of new found energy nearly took my breath away.

A feeling welled up from deep within me when I realized that,

This is WORKING!

I felt a surge of hope in that moment I don't believe I have felt since that day. I had risked everything. I went out on such an out stretched limb, almost dangling in midair some days for this procedure and here it is already working!

I am here for a purpose and that purpose is to grow into a mountain, not shrink to a grain of sand. Henceforth, I will apply all my efforts to become the highest mountain of all and I will strain my potential until it screams for mercy.

Og Mandino

You May Need A Guide

When I was 15 I climbed Mt. Rainier. It is a majestic active volcano southeast of Seattle Washington, it can be seen from just about anywhere and it is a beautiful mountain. I had always had a sense of awe when it came to it. It is 14,411 feet tall making it the 3rd largest mountain in the United States. It was as imposing to me as my later goal of walking again.

What mirrored each other in this case is I couldn't reach my goal with either mountain without a guide. A guide is someone who knows more than you and you must trust and rely upon this guide with your life. In the case of climbing Mt Rainier that is a literal case.

I didn't have a clue about learning how to walk either. I wouldn't know the first thing to work on or if there was even an order to that chaos. If I hadn't trained for a year to learn new skill sets to climb a mountain I could have died.

We spent the following year preparing for this climb. None of us had done anything more than hiking in the nearby mountains so we learned about the different components that we needed in order to accomplish this. We learned about rope teams, ice axes, self-arrest and many other important things in order to safely climb this mountain.

The day finally came to depart and it was a beautiful Seattle day, no rain! Actually it was a gorgeous blue sky day. We reached base camp, Camp Muir at 10,000 feet and settled in to rest and sleep for the afternoon and evening. We set out at 2 a.m. in order to summit and be able to come back before it got too warm and too late.

We left Camp Muir and hiked along the base of some rock outcroppings to a ridge which we had to traverse. Once we were over this ridge the pathway took us into a large glacier field when the first major stop we had to do was right before we crossed an ice fall. This area was huge and even though we couldn't see in the dark we knew what we were facing. Large stacks of ice as big as or bigger than a house were littered all down this steep area of the mountain. It is so dangerous that in 1983 11 climbers died when an avalanche occurred that buried them. All they ever found, we were told, was a glove. Many of our group were having equipment troubles and were going to be forced to turn back. The 6 of 16 that remained were each asked a question as we huddled around each other determining who could and wished to go on. We were each asked, do you wish to continue.

This question has the ability to haunt you. You see your life flash before your eyes. The most dangerous portion of the climb was ahead and there would be no shame in saying no. But if you said yes, then you would be so outside of your comfort zone that you will be scared out of your mind. You were committed.

I took a deep breath in and I answered, Yes, I would continue!

We each took stock in our gear, crampons, ropes (we were put into teams of four, all roped together for safety). We booked it across the bottom of the ice fall and reached the bottom of Disappointed Cleaver and let out a huge sigh. We had crossed below the falls silently as the slightest sound could trigger an avalanche. Disappointment Cleaver is a large rock cliff that stands out from the mountain. It was probably 800-1000 feet high. The path, if you could call it a path, was the little rock avalanches you see trailing down a steep cliff or trail. That is what we used as our path. It was slow climbing since we had our crampons on and they are a little tricky going up loose rock but we couldn't have had much solid footing without them. Midway up I remember taking a rest and taking my gloves off to warm my hands in the steam vents billowing out from the mountain.

Once we got to the top we saw the most amazing sunrise I have ever witnessed. Imagine a sunrise that stretched from Canada to Oregon. I do not have the words to this day of how beautiful this was to witness.

From there we continued our hike up and even had to cross over a large ice bridge. Once we made the summit most of us continued on to what's called the true summit. Most that climb Mt Rainier actually do not go on to the true summit. In order to make the true summit we had to climb down to the crater and walk across it and up the other side. I later learned that we were walking over 200 feet of snow and ice. We signed the log book at the summit indicating we had done it. We could see Canada, Oregon and even the Pacific Ocean and so far into Eastern Washington it might have been Idaho! This is one of the most memorable moments in my life.

Before this would I have attempted to climb this mountain? Could I have? No to both. I needed a guide in order to understand how to climb this mountain, know the path, understand and prepare for the dangers.

Just as I needed a guide to climb Mt Rainier I needed a guide to teach me how to walk again. I had no idea the proper path to do so. I didn't know anything that might have helped me get there. The guides would be my physical therapists. They knew what order to go in, they knew how to push me further and further than I would have or could have on my own. I needed them for their knowledge and expertise. They were also my biggest cheerleaders and would push me the hardest when they knew I had more in me to give.

Each of us will need a guide at some point in our lives. We could always use the moral support and count on a cheerleader in our corner. I know it helped me more than I could ever put into words.

I knew when I got back home after the stem cell transplant I would need a guide, a physical therapist as it turns out, is who I made an appointment with upon returning home.

Wanting something is not enough. You must hunger for it. Your motivation must be absolutely compelling in order to overcome the obstacles that will invariably come your way.

Les Brown

The Other Side Of Hard Work Was My Goal

In March 2005 I met with a physical therapist, Jason, a few weeks after arriving home. The first thing he asked me was what my goal was, I replied, "Walking". As he was writing this down I said to him "Oh yea, if you don't kick my ass I'm going to kick yours!" He dropped the pen and looked up at me. I lifted my left hand into the air above my knee about even with my head and said "There is nothing in the way of me walking so just do what it takes to do your job." Regrets for the language but that is what I said and I said it to make sure we were on the same page from the beginning. I needed to make sure I was putting my trust into someone who knew exactly what my goal was and felt he could carry me through to the results I desired.

I'm not sure what he thought of me at the time but I am sure he wanted to kick my butt after that exchange! We soon became friends as I did whatever he and another therapist named Stephanie asked me to perform. I would give them hell every time but I would never not do what they asked. I was going to walk again. Nothing would stand in my way. Not even my own body.

In the beginning, I could move my right big toe a quarter of an inch is all. I couldn't even swing my leg as it dangled over the edge of a raised table. I was going from paralyzed to walking and I went about it like an ignorant child. I was determined. I had a goal. And I had no idea if I was going to reach this goal but I wasn't about to go down without giving it everything from my soul.

It's amazing what you can get used to. I remember the first time they had me up in some leg braces and since it had been some time since I had stood on my legs the standing perspective was so foreign and my spatial view so skewed that I felt dizzy with only a few feet elevation change. I had to focus on other parts of the room to obtain a spot on which to focus, then I could balance myself and gain some equilibrium before I could take a step. Once I figured that out, walking from then on gained momentum. This applied especially when I began walking outside. I needed to focus on something solid and steady like a tree or rock or even the curb as my focal point, otherwise I couldn't gain that equilibrium and therefore couldn't walk without becoming dizzy. Over time this became less and less needed since I started to become more used to being on my feet. To this day I don't need to check with a steady solid object indoors and only every so often outdoors.

I worked hard at regaining this common ability so many times before but this was the first time where I could actually take steps on my own without any aids. I actually could lift my legs and move them forward under my own strength. This was both exciting and exhilarating to me and was exciting to know things were coming back. This was real vindication for me.

The real battle during all of this (and still is to this day) is the mental realization that I do not have to use the chair as much anymore. I can stand, I can walk, and I can do more and more of both and stay longer out of the chair. Sometimes it is difficult to remember the 'I can' in all of this. This goes back to how I was raised and all the successful mantra's that were not instilled in me. I think the fact that it is still somewhat difficult for me to remember "I can" indicates how tough it is to overturn those negative lessons many of us have been taught. They are very powerful and can undo years of work in an instant. I can only keep on achieving further victories and I hope in time that I will never doubt myself again. It is a journey of self-discovery. Reworking my mind around what have been lifelong battles in the mind. I keep fighting those battles in hopes of winning the war. They are harder to fight some days than others but you just have to keep putting one foot in front of the other going forward one step at a time. And keep telling yourself "I'm possible!"

It is strange how with all that I have been through I still revert back to what is more familiar to me, I have worked hard to replace the old affirmations with new stronger, positive ones. Those continuous victories help in that task. They aid in building a stronger more firm foundation that will support me as I continue to heal. It is important to strengthen your foundation positively and as often as you can. It is difficult at first but with each seemingly small victory is another layer built up on your foundation.

My foundation in the beginning of this healing journey was built upon the idea that I could overcome these diseases and that I would walk again. The stem cell transplant was a layer. The physical therapy was a layer. The reaction to the physical stimuli was yet another layer. As I add these layers I find that my legs respond in kind. If I push them they grow stronger and more agile. As I become more agile I begin to look like an adult who has walked all his life instead of the struggling 18 month old child figuring things out for the first time.

Within 18 months of the twice a week sessions with my physical therapists I was able to walk 300 feet with the use of two canes. It was amazing to go that distance. It was exhausting, of course, but I was walking! Who cares about a little tiredness right? The most difficult thing to overcome (and it has always been the most difficult thing to overcome) is ME.

I am the greatest hurdle to my success. If I cannot fake it till I make it I won't make it at all. In order to walk again one needs one thing, faith. Faith is an action word, without it there is no achievement in any field. Faith by its very nature calls upon us to put some work into it. It doesn't matter what the "it" is. If we are not willing to place one foot in front of the other day in and day out you will get exactly

NO WHERE.

I started nowhere so why not go somewhere?

Most of what I see in America these days is instant gratification. If I had that mindset I would have given up a long time ago. Learning something new is always difficult. That's what makes it new. If it were old you wouldn't be thinking it is tough to do. It wouldn't even be on your mind. Walking again has taken a lot longer than it could have because, as much as I wanted to walk and willed myself to be able to obtain it, I still didn't have the faith component down. It wasn't what made up my core belief system yet. That has taken a long while to understand that it was missing. Once I was cut from physical therapy, I floundered for a while because I hadn't instilled this into my belief system. Inside I was still a mine field. I still needed that outside influence to keep me going until I could literally stand up on my own both emotionally and physically.

The false emotional thinking, the bad programming as a child instilled in me the notion that I wasn't worth it. I wasn't able to overcome anything because it was impossible. I was unworthy of anything positive or uplifting. I don't do amazing things because, who am I to do amazing things?

Who am I NOT to? I had to ask myself this question and when there was no satisfactory answer I had to then believe that I was indeed worthy and I had a positive potential and that I could.

Who ever thought it would help someone to not get their hopes up or to not allow their imagination to take them to the edge of disappointment are the losers of this world. They are they who have placed these limitations upon others because they imposed limitations upon themselves. They cannot stand someone else to be more successful than themselves so they instill a discouragement program into others. Our whole society is built upon this lie.

It is time we stop this limited mindset and just allow ourselves and especially allow others to succeed in whatever the endeavor. Who knows, all of us might be surprised where our victories show up!

Physically healing forced me to face these untruths I had grown up with. If it meant something to me I needed to change the stories in my head. Learning to walk again has been the catalyst to positive change that I didn't know I needed. I needed to understand and to comprehend that I most sincerely could do whatever I wanted. I really could be anything I wanted to be. It is a simple thought but it isn't easy to get outside our heads long enough to make that declaration to ourselves and the Universe. Once we become clear on this then we can become clear on our intentions.

I intended to walk. I never set out to change perceptions or to challenge the medical society with the result of those actions. I only intended to walk again. In so doing I have learned I have done something no one else has in the world. I have become 'that guy.' I don't want to be 'that guy' that breaks all the rules so you have permission to realize you can too! But apparently I am.

Defying doctors has brought me here. For years no doctor would acknowledge my statement that I will walk again. While none would verbalize that it wasn't going to happen they would ignore my statements when I said I would. Defying what was in their eyes as "impossible" has allowed me to define what is possible for me. Therein lays the message of my life.

Impossible is somebody else's opinion.

I AM Possible is my opinion.

The opinion you believe is the reality you achieve.

Until we can receive with an open heart, we're never really giving with an open heart. When we attach judgment to receiving help, we knowingly or unknowingly attach judgment to giving help.

Brené Brown

Accept Help From Others – (Im)Possible Principle

There's a reason that even speakers, coaches or mentors have coaches or mentors to help them through rough times and even the good times. In the good times, no matter how honest you are with yourself you will favor yourself rather than push through those bad times when you might need an outsider to push you beyond what you thought was possible, or what your vision allowed you to see.

I think of my trainer Surba Tucker. He and I were brought together at just the right time to be able to push me further along in healing and walking than I was looking for. I was upright and walking a little bit, wasn't that enough? As it turns out no. I am miles beyond what I thought was possible even for me. He pushed me and prodded me and essentially made me stand up and be more. With that foundation of "I can" I have gone further in other areas than I even thought possible on my own.

He saw a vision of what was possible even before I could. He saw what I was capable of and took me along that path. He believed in me long before I could. That kept me going. That support helped me while I was forming new belief systems about myself and what was possible for me. I needed to form this opinion for me because he wasn't about to do the work for me. I needed to show up for myself and Surba has been a lifesaver for me that way.

It's okay to need others along your path, it's not a sign of weakness but rather a show of strength and trust to allow another to step in and make up for your inadequacies. We all have them and we all will need help. Suck up the pride and take that step, you won't regret it.

Life's challenges are not supposed to paralyze you, they're supposed to help you discover who you are.

Johnson Reagon

Healing Isn't Always Beautiful

I did it. I was learning to walk. In fact, I could walk quite well. That's it right? I recovered from paralysis. I can handle this level of walking and be fine about it the rest of my life. This was what I settled for once I was able to walk a bit. I settled.

For years I justified not working towards the overall ability to not need the wheelchair ever again. I was afraid. I was afraid of what I didn't understand. In a subtle way the wheelchair became my identity. I wasn't beholden to it but on a subliminal emotional level I was attached to it as a part of my identity. It actually pains me to see this in writing. I settled.

What no one was able to prepare me for was the confusion and inability to fully understand that my mindset wasn't changing with my recovery. No one had been here before so how anyone could have known the issue with recovering from paralysis and the stem cell transplant? I didn't even understand it. In fact, for years I couldn't verbalize the issue I felt welling within me. Causing me to lash out at the world and become quite frankly, unsupportable. Friends would respond to my outburst that "Healing sucks" with the proverbial "But you're walking right?" I couldn't verbalize it then but it wasn't about the walking. It wasn't in fact about the stem cell transplant. It was about healing. I didn't know what that was for some years to come.

During those years I was suffering from PTSD (Post-Traumatic Stress Disorder). This is a specific set of symptoms we usually closely associate with war and returning veterans. It is a terrible set of symptoms that the sufferer usually doesn't realize he/her is suffering from. The point is traumatic stress, trauma comes in many forms and varieties and there is no telling how we will react to different scenarios. I even saw a therapist and proved that I had every single symptom. But there was no true treatment that helps so I sort of taunted him with this revelation.

I now realize that the abusive family background I grew up in set the foundation for this. When I left home I ended up leaving the state to get away from such a negative state of being with the mindset that I could now choose my own way of choosing and living and I would be fine. I thought wrong. While I may have left the source of abuse the effects of it were within me. Deep within me. I didn't know it at the time but I was a ticking bomb that needed to let the pressure go. That came to light a little when my parents announced they were getting divorced. I thought, "Ten years too late, but thanks for trying."

For some months after this announcement a flood of emotion and hurt and anger came rushing back to the surface. I was so overwhelmed with it I could hardly eat for weeks and weeks. I was very physical and for a time I lost a belt loop a week. I was wasting away from the reemergence of these negative thoughts, emotions, and experiences. Yet, I couldn't properly express words or sentences to even describe what I was feeling. All I knew was I felt, I hurt, and the pain was excruciating.

It wasn't but a year and a half later that I experienced the first symptoms of numbness and paralysis. I had left the source of all this pain but what I didn't realize is I carried it all within me. It was buried pretty deep and I ignored it, thinking I will be okay because I left and I was on my own happily making my own decisions. Or was I?

That background was dictating my every move and I didn't realize it. I was living and making decisions based upon this angst, hurt, and anger and it was going to kill me if I kept it in. It did try to kill me. I nearly died several times during the subsequent illness. Twice I was in serious car accidents where I was inches from death, and should have died. Which is fitting because deep down and it took years to acknowledge this, I did indeed wish to die. Any dream I had as a child would be of me being swallowed by rushing water going down a storm drain, swept away to a dark abyss.

It was the only reoccurring dream I ever had growing up and I haven't had a dream I remember since the time I was about 12. Funny that is when the abuse stepped up once my father became ill. I had wanted to die for years. I felt unimportant and a throw away. In a way that was a part of the reason the symptoms began. I propelled those emotions into my very being. The foundational piece for all of this was I was acting out the very abuse I grew up in only it was self-abuse. I turned it towards myself because my own self-worth was next to nothing.

Imagine how I felt after going through those seven years of symptoms ranging from paralysis to death. After experiencing so much for so long I thrust myself into a study. A study mind you. An experiment I volunteered to be a Guinea Pig with no guarantee of success. With nearly three months of being poked and prodded and put through unimaginable hell I emerged. But what emerged?

Years further of very regular long trips and poking and prodding during checkups. As I began to heal physically from the paralysis I saw my goals being met with success. There was a brighter future beginning and I thought, "Once I am walking again everything is going to be fine." During this time frame is when I began to become accepting of the mediocrity that became my life. I was okay with being able to walk a few hundred feet, that's all I needed, right? As long as I could place my wheelchair in my vehicle and get up a few stairs from time to time I would be just fine. Best of both worlds I told myself. I told myself that lie for years. And I began to believe it more and more until one evening. I was on a couch talking to my girlfriend at the time and you know when you actually hear what you're saying? It caused me to stop mid-sentence and push her off my lap. I grabbed her lap top to type in what I had just said. I said that I was healing physically in order to heal emotionally from the stuff that led to me getting sick in the first place. Wow. Where did that even come from? I was dumbfounded and shocked to the core. I basically was saying that my childhood of abuse was the cause of my diseases. I was blaming them for what happened to me physically and that it was time to address the core issue.

I hated God that day. I kept saying that to myself and to Him both silently in my head and out loud in outbursts of disgust. Wasn't this enough? Hadn't I done enough by walking again? I hated Him for at least 6 to 8 months after that. How much more could I take? I didn't know if I could handle being told that there was more I needed to do. I was exhausted. I was so worn out by this time that I didn't, no, I couldn't think about having to go through more. I needed a break or I was going to break.

I broke. I lost interest in trying anymore and it was during this time I began to realize I was undergoing the symptoms of PTSD. I also began to understand the significance of healing and what that really means. Healing isn't a one-time thing and you move on. It is a process. It is sometimes a short process or a long drawn out one depending on the severity of the thing that one is recovering from.

Balance.

Healing is balance and nothing more. I was so incredibly out of balance that it took something as severe as the years of paralysis for it to manifest itself. It showed up big and I needed to return the favor or it was going to beat me down and perhaps destroy me. But I needed to try.

One thing you need to know about me is I may destroy myself but I will never allow something or someone to destroy me. I will fight. I have this place within me that won't allow anything outside of myself to destroy or hurt me. I will fight to the death and death was what I courted for many years. I decided somewhere along this path that I was worth fighting for. If I was going to die from all this I wasn't going down without a fight. I would fight for me. For I was possible.

It was over three years ago since that epiphany occurred. I have worked hard to not only distance myself from the abusive past and the extremely damaging effects of the ensuing disease processes. I worked hard to learn to understand that none of this was my fault and that it was things done to me, they were not me. They may have led to my becoming the person I am today; however, they in no way defined me. This was the beginning of three years of learning the broad damaging effects of abuse and negative emotions. This led me to more fully understand the connectivity of negative thoughts, actions and disease. My physical disease was a direct manifestation of the background of abuse. I could end it. Powerful thought right? It was within my power and CHOICE to choose how I wanted to live the rest of my life, free from that past.

I chose to have this manifest itself through my continued efforts to walk more. I began to ponder why I hadn't yet shown up for me. I showed up for my physical therapists, I was showing up for my personal trainer but I hadn't shown up for the most important person in this puzzle. Me. This thought took me by surprise. I wasn't really pushing myself to my stated goal of walking because I hadn't shown up for me because I was still caught in that old mindset of abuse and feeling worthless. I began showing up at the gym for myself from that moment. An interesting thing happened. I was able to go from walking a tenth of a mile on the treadmill to walking a full mile within 9 months. Within that same time period I went from leg pressing 100 pounds 15 times to pressing 240 pounds and have even pressed 307 pounds 15 times since then. My body responded when my thoughts turned to action. That action instilled my belief today that not only am I possible but I am also worth it. My legs since then have done everything I have asked of them and then some. When I showed up I gave myself permission to throw away the old mindset and create a new one. It is one based upon possibilities. I have set no limits and I have surpassed every goal I ever thought probable.

In March of 2015, I climbed the stairs of a 24 story building here in Salt Lake City. When I set a goal it will now become reality because

I have seen through the lie that it cannot be done. Setting the goal. Creating a reality of achievement list, what will it take to achieve this goal work sheet? I write down the steps it is going to take to achieve the goal. I break it up into bite size pieces. I then focus on only that step until it is achieved then I move to the next. I only go in order from there. Where there is order there is a process of achievement. Once I achieve the goal I take the time to relish in that achievement. I don't rob myself of the enjoyment anymore.

With each goal reached I place another layer to my foundation. Each and every success creates a stronger foundation. With a strong foundation there isn't anything one cannot achieve. Building it up is the key. It takes each and every little victory, no matter the size, to take you from nothing to something in no time. Alright, it has taken me 10 years to get this far in my walking goal but no matter the size of the goal the process is still the same. Build up your foundation a victory at a time and don't get caught up in the time it takes to reach it. The time shouldn't matter. Write down the reality of achievement list and set it to action. Time frame goals sometimes are a detriment to your understanding of achievement and enjoyment. They sometimes get in the way of enjoying the path. Enjoy the steps and relish in each and every victory. You deserve it.

I deserved to learn this lesson. It took a while to understand that I was indeed building a foundation. I at first needed to rely upon the vision and strength of other people. Once I felt strong enough to stand on my own I then realized it was time to show up for myself. My success is based upon the foundation of other people's principles until I learned what my own principles were. I feel my true success only began once I was able to show up for myself. One I formed my own vision and inner strength I felt ready to conquer anything.

Over time my mindset has been able to slowly grasp gratitude and my ability to be appreciative of all that I have experienced; no matter the negative framing I would place it. I was indeed grateful and still am on many levels for these experiences for it has shown me that no matter the situation there is a way out. No matter what it is there is a path out. And you CHOOSE what it is.

What a wonderful lesson for me to learn. Despite my family's best efforts to destroy me, despite life's best efforts to destroy me and despite my best efforts to destroy myself I have FOUND myself. And I have found I rather like myself and what I stand for.

I can now be most grateful for these wonderful lessons that I am okay and no one defines me. I define myself and that is the greatest gift I have ever received. The stem cell transplant was a catalyst to a certain level of healing. Walking again was its own level of healing and understanding that I could indeed overcome something quite impossible in the world's eyes. My own exploration of healing on an emotional level was kooky at first and a bit of weird voodoo hoodoo but I have emerged the other side exactly where I had pictured myself years ago.

I knew on the other side of work which came in the form of blood sweat and tears that what I wanted was worth it. I knew that it would take a lot of work. I knew it would hurt. But I also knew it was worth it to me. So it is in everything we each choose to do in this life. If the end result is worth the effort required it doesn't matter how impossible others may view it. If you believe it is possible you will achieve it because only you know and understand the reasons why it is important for you to achieve it. And you will be able to make it happen.

I hope any of you reading this will realize that you are indeed possible. That no matter the issues you are facing there is a pathway out of that suffering. Whether it is physical, emotional, mental, or spiritual there is a way out. It may take time, it may take equipment, and it can and should take the help of friends and loved ones to help show you a different way. The bottom line is there is always a way out of the impossible. For the possible hasn't been tried yet. Keep looking. It will find you in the end if it is what you truly wish for.

I only wish more people would see the solution to their problems this way. There is too much depression, anxiety and feelings of worthlessness out there. IF only we all could see the possibilities what impossibility would we accomplish today.

I am not easily discouraged. I readily visualized myself as overcoming obstacles, winning out over setbacks, achieving impossible objectives.

Bruce Lee

Belief Is A Dream And Faith Is Action

Do you work harder than everybody else? Those that work harder usually deserve all that they get as a result. Most of the time we don't see what they do behind the scenes and we tend to judge based upon that assumption. All of us have things that we do behind the scenes and they are for us to know. Putting into the work needed to gain a new skill for example is necessary if you wish to get out of a situation that your current mindset created.

If this is the case then you need to change your thinking otherwise you will never outdo yourself and get out of that situation. Learn that new skill or do the work out differently to gain something new. When we do this we expand our mindsets, our goals and our outlook. Sometimes we might not even know what we did differently, especially when it comes to mindset. Most of us are trapped in that space between our ears and if we stay there too long we accomplish exactly that, nothing but a thought and perhaps a dream. To put that thought into an actionable goal we need to bring some action to the effort.

Faith is an active word so we must DO something to gain from that faith. What we gain after the experience of faith is knowledge. Replacing faith with knowledge ought to be in each of our goals. By turning that belief into faith and that faith into knowledge we find ourselves upon such a solid foundation that nothing will be able to knock us off of it. We gain self confidence in this exact manner. Self-confidence is foundational experiences that beef up our belief in ourselves and in our abilities. When I doubted myself or my potential I doubted what I had already accomplished and made it into a mockery of sorts. I had already accomplished so much, yet I couldn't see the forest through the trees. I was blinded to the future because I could only focus on that past. I was distracted enough to begin believing my self-doubts and not my successes.

These periods of time negated all that I had worked up to. I threw things away because of this lack of self-belief. What a waste to keep doing that over and over again. I was still in my old mindset, not seeing I had already won. I had accomplished much but I chose instead to throw it all away. I didn't know this at the time but I threw away great forward motion for mediocrity.

How many times have you stopped mid stride or mid goal distracted by your doubts and other non-essential distractions? If you're like me probably a lot. Staying focused on not only the top of the hill where I would usually rest, I was taught by my coaches to focus instead upon something no one else was willing to focus on. By instilling this work ethic and the mindset and willingness to work harder than anybody else a great foundational principle was born. Be willing to do more than everybody else to set yourself apart from the crowd. Truly successful people do this. We see it in many football athletes, baseball, boxing and just about any other sport. The ones on top do things out of the public eye that delineates them from you and me. They work out more, they incorporate seemingly unconnected things together to establish a broader more firm foundation of strength and endurance.

That is why they are the best. They don't do it for anybody but themselves. It means that much to their self-belief and awareness. They absolutely have to do more than everybody else was willing to go to my physical therapist that first day and lay it out what I was willing to do and what I expected out of him. I put it out there and both Jason and Stephanie met and even surpassed my challenge. They were able to surpass my challenge because their personality wouldn't allow anything less. I had met my match and then some. I continually meet these personality types in my life. My personal trainer and friend Surba Tucker is exactly like this. He has high expectations for himself and that translates into a high expectation for his clients. What is awesome about he and I is that when he puts out the challenge for a new movement or exercise I meet it head on. When I, on my own time, exceed where we are strength and endurance wise I share what I've done and he then one ups me.

Back and forth for almost 5 years we have silently been playing this game of one up man ship. It is what pushes me forward. He also has an innate ability to see your abilities long before you do. His vision and how he fashions his workouts for you to meet that expectation is quite literally art. It is an unbelievable talent that few possess.

Whenever I have met his expectations and have sat there in disbelief that I was able to do this type of exercise for the first time his response is always you were ready. That progression was natural and to him was expected. While in my head I am exclaiming, are you serious? I have never done that in 17 years, or I haven't felt that part of my legs in that long. He expected it. I should also but mentally it has been difficult to grasp how much I have been gaining back. As far forward as my expectations were I have never expected all that I am able to do lately.

Due to my friendship with him, I have had to raise my expectations to a higher standard. My self-awareness has risen to a height I have never been at. Now that I know this I can't go backwards. Yet this is what many of us do when we have reached or surpassed our goals and we even do it before we reach our goal. We self-sabotage those efforts. When we do this we hold doubt in higher esteem than our potential and we automatically sell ourselves short. We have most likely stopped just short of amazing things happening to us. I used to do this years ago when I was let go from physical therapy to work out on my own. I couldn't keep the momentum going because my personal foundation wasn't yet setup. I was relying on everybody else's efforts and not believing in my own possibilities. It's not like I doubted, I just never gave it a thought. How sad that is to admit. As much as I wanted to walk and had shown exceptional progress I had never transplanted that success into a self-belief that I could actually do this and I could do it on my own and I could even succeed at it.

It's been the hardest part of healing to be honest. To translate the very visible successes into fundamental belief systems that could then propel me onto a newer and higher plane of thinking. I keptmyself in a lower mindset because my foundation was still based upon the lies of my childhood. I couldn't yet grasp my importance to not only myself, to my friends, to strangers who hear my story,and to the world. I at the time couldn't accept that past. Mentally and emotionally I was still running from it. And if I am running from it how can I face it and overcome it?

Once I started facing my past, to acknowledge it, I was able to see a path that led me around it. Soon it began to lead me from it. Now I am so detached from that foundation of lies that I can never accept them into my heart or mind again. I have been opened to new possibilities which have lead me to a higher level of thinking not only about myself, my abilities but my future and what I see as possible. Quite frankly there is nothing holding me back anymore. The only thing really holding me back is the fact I haven't thought of it yet.

When a friend suggested I do a stair climb challenge it took me about 6 minutes to conclude that I must meet the uncomfortable challenge, but if I put a plan together I could possibly make it to the top. The top was the 24 story Wells Fargo building in Salt Lake City. The event is a fundraiser for Huntsman Cancer Institute. I prepared by mapping out how long I had to accomplish this goal and then I set about writing down what it is I needed to be able to physically do before I could feel good about making it to the top. Six weeks later was the day. I took a deep breath in and began climbing. There were a lot of people doing this and there was a lot of encouragement the whole day. I had two news stations there to film and do stories. Soooooooo.... I had to show up and I had better make it worth their while!

Don't let what you cannot do interfere with what you can do.

John Wooden

The Missing Ingredient

My book is titled Impossible, Or So They Said, my original title was Start at the Finish Line. It began by including starting, but in order to capture the urgency of beginning my task and subsequently your task we must just START NOW.

Do not hesitate. When one hesitates one finds excuses and excuses put off what you know you need to be working on. It is the urgency to act that separates the dreamers from the doers. Many people dream.

I dream. If I want to keep the dream alone I merely need to keep dreaming. If I wish to make the dream a reality then I must act upon that dream. Wish I shoulda, woulda, coulda becomes the inner mantra of the dreamer after it becomes too late to act upon the dream.

To start the finish line means to just take a step away from where you are currently. It really doesn't matter the destination. It matters that you begin the journey in the first place. How many of us know of a dreamer. Stuck in the wishing. And therefore stuck in the now, and perhaps a lot of yesterday? In some areas of my life I am that stuck dreamer. I am a dreamer. I can admit that.

Sometimes the dreaming comes along a lot earlier than the means of achieving the dream are available. This is okay. There are perhaps many steps to get you prepared to act on achievement of the dream. Mental preparation is the first step.

I dreamed for years of walking again. I wouldn't have the stem cell opportunity for 7 years. I dreamed of walking. I angered doctors with that dream. I am sure I bored many friends with that dream. BUT, it was MY dream and no one could take that away.

Along the way during those 7 years I kept trying to walk again. No matter how desperate the prognosis looked I was always in physical therapy being taught how to walk. How to use my legs. It was constant. I was consistently in rehab for those 7 years because my dream meant that much to me. I would walk again someday. I knew it deep in my heart. It was a core belief of mine that never wavered. Therefore I kept at it. No matter how many times I was knocked down, I got right back up; it was so deeply ingrained in me to push that I couldn't not try to achieve my goal.

Even though the first step is the hardest one I literally stayed on the first step for 7 years until the opportunity came. The catalyst was stem cells. Perhaps it was the missing piece. Did it really help heal me from the inside out so that I could indeed walk again or was it such a powerful motivator that that was all I needed mentally in order to make the gains that I did. I don't have an answer to that. I feel it was a little of both actually.

Perhaps it was just the boost I needed to jump start the health from the inside out and enough of a catalyst that my mind focused on it just long enough to achieve little victories spurring me on to achieve further victories until I am where I am today.

While each victory was achieved and laid upon the last victory soon I had amassed a very stable foundation to what is now an expectation of full use of my legs. I fully expect to use the wheelchair less and less over the course of time. It is achievable. It is within the realm of possibility.

The point is why waste so much energy thinking of beginning and why not just stand up and take a step? You will inevitably change direction but tell me in what area of life do you not change direction because of a gain, or new insight. Course correction happens all on its own. You don't have to necessarily think of everything right now. You just have to act upon it, right now. Had I waited and wondered how long it would take to walk again and how it would happen etc. I would still be confined to my wheelchair and not spending more and more time out of it. I took the first step which was to ask for help in teaching me this skill I hadn't needed to learn since I was a small child.

Upon requesting the help I needed from those who specialized in helping others with this type of goal I showed up. Showing up accomplishes over half of our goals and objectives in this life. Many things happen when we show up. How committed to our goal are we? What are we willing to do to achieve it? The way I put it is this. If what I want is over there and I want it badly enough, the "stuff" in between me and that goal achievement will not deter me. No matter the blood sweat and tears that are shed, I will do anything in my power to make it happen. This is the "work" part of goal achievement.

Why does work deter you from achieving your goals? Too hard? Too painful? How hard and painful is regret?

If what you want on the other side of work is worth it to you those are not complaints, those are powerful motivators to your change. When you believe these things to the core you will achieve them.

If I wanted to use the "it's too hard" complaint then I would not be worthy of the ability to walk. Life is already difficult for most if not all of us. Why point it out all the time. That is focusing on the wrong portion of the solution. Too hard was assumed consciously. I knew it would be tough. I had 7 years to glimpse how difficult it would be. I went all in knowing full well that it would be difficult. I didn't have to complain about it. That is a waste of energy.

Instead I was buoyed by every small or large victory along the way. They justified my outrageous goal of walking again. Every single victory made the "work" part justified. It made each tough day worth it.

I got over those tough days rather quickly as I kept moving forward towards the next little victory that would keep my momentum. As long as I had momentum I ensured myself further victories. I kept putting more effort into walking and I got more in return. If I pushed it a little harder then I got a little further. The more I put into it the more I got out of it. As long as I stayed focused on that equal exchange then I fueled the effort needed to continue. I began to feed my own efforts with my own results. As I did so I learned about perpetual motion. I was in a perpetual action of giving and receiving. As long as I didn't interrupt that symphony I would continue to see the sweet sounds of this music I was creating.

I have achieved all that I felt I would achieve, and more. I am being blown away every day now. I have gone on way past any goal I ever had when it came to my concept of walking again. I drive without hand controls on my vehicle. I sometimes leave my home without my wheelchair. I go to restaurants and walk in. I walk out and drive home all without my wheelchair. I can walk a mile on the treadmill. I can jump on the elliptical machine for 20-25 minutes now. I can climb 24 stories. I can walk over 100feet while carrying two 35 pound dumbbells that is 70 pounds! There is no end to my progress and I am now am using a walker when I am outside my home. I am continually blowing my mind.

What I have done is so crazy to me that I often have to pinch myself if this is real or not. I mean, the wheelchair is pretty much a support vehicle now. It isn't my only support anymore. And that concept is still rather mind-boggling to me. I know I have worked at this for 10 years now but I am constantly in a state of disbelief at what I am able to accomplish. Truly I am.

I think I am still in a state of disbelief because I have along the way learned about gratitude. I am so grateful for the progress I have made because I showed up for myself and kept on applying the effort needed in order to accomplish this impossible goal of walking.

This leads me to the second part, Impossible and I'm Possible are two of the greatest deterrents to progress and yet they are the only two reasons anything ever gets accomplished. Focus and perspective are very similar words in this case. Whatever your focus is you will obtain that.

Perspective gives you focus. If you perceive that something is impossible then you will find out that yes indeed it is impossible. When you change your perspective to "perhaps there is a way to achieve this" and overcome any belief that something is impossible then the focus changes and therefore the effort becomes more intense on finding a way around the impossible.

Every once in a while you will hear in the news about someone doing something once thought impossible. It wasn't impossible, someone hadn't figured it out yet is all. And so it goes that impossible is somebody else's opinion. The problem is that just about EVERYBODY believes it.

So, therefore it becomes impossible. It will stay that way until someone comes along and says you know, if I do it this way, or go this route or make a machine that does this instead then.... See how easy it is to overcome the crowd? Thinking differently than society or the crowd is what gives us hope. It gives permission for the rest of us to think like they do and the once impossible becomes every day until that new glass ceiling shatters and a new high achieved.

The problem and the blessing of thinking I'm Possible is that there are too many people in society that do not believe that they are possible. I am only beginning to feel I'm Possible. I have never attached the most important component to walking and overcoming something thought impossible and that is: believing I'M Possible. Overcoming somebody else's opinion is an easy step, but, overcoming ME?

That is a hornet's nest of issues.

For me this got into the abusive upbringing I survived. I was constantly pounded with conflicting messages that would tell me I could do anything I wanted with don't do it that way or you can't do it that way or accomplish this. I was so beat down on an emotional level that any thought of positivity when it came to me and I would

121

run from that thought or quickly bury it. It literally caused me to quit thinking that way. It is a daily thing to overcome such a heavy and negative mindset that has prevented me from believing in myself. I have detested myself for so long that it is like a foreign invader in my life to even feel that I am anywhere near possible. I constantly have to shut down those negative thoughts and focus on what I have accomplished and change the story I tell myself.

We are all Possible my friends.

Every. Single. One. Of. Us.

Take a minute to look back on your life and think of all that you have accomplished. If you just take a minute and list those things that have come to your mind you would be a little surprised at how long that list becomes. It only takes a little remembering for us to find that we have each done amazing things to get this far in life. As a society we focus so much on tomorrow we forget all about yesterday and barely live in today so we don't notice we have the ability to make such an impact upon this world.

I have to switch my focus to better appreciate all that I have done and how far I have come. It is easy to get caught up in the whirlwind of making sure you are working towards the 'this and that' of tomorrow to forget to LIVE today and remember yesterday with fondness instead of disdain or forgetfulness.

Remember all that you have done to get here and you will have a solid foundation of gratitude and be able to appreciate all that comes your way. This leads me to the rest of the title. One step at a time. Every step will lead you closer to that which you focus on. What impossible thing have you locked from making any progress on? We all have them. One of my big ones was writing this book.

Who would want to read about my life I asked myself all too often. What do I have to say to the world that the world would listen? This kind of mindset is a shrinking mindset and it isn't a positive one at all. Each and every one of us has something to contribute to the betterment of the world. I began attacking the goal of writing this book by mindlessly writing. I needed a brain purge and this allowed me to vomit words onto a page which allowed me inside my own head. The more I did that as an exercise the more I found my voice. I may not be able to speak this way verbally but I can communicate my thoughts via the written word much more eloquently than in speech. The more I did this the more I realized I may have an ability to write a book after all. As I gained small victory after victory I gained enough of a foundation to be able to realize that the message I needed to write wasn't available anywhere else and that I needed to share it with you.

What is my goal in having you read my words? For you to find your own. Perhaps, like me, your actions speak louder than words. Now go and ACT out your story. The world needs to see you. If you're able to write then the world needs to HEAR you. And if your ability is to speak then the world needs to SEE you speak your truths.

The one thing the world is missing?

YOU

Made in the USA
San Bernardino, CA
13 November 2015